AIDS in the Heartland

AIDS in the Heartland
How Unlikely Coalitions Created a Blueprint for LGBTQ Politics

Katie Batza

The University of North Carolina Press CHAPEL HILL

© 2025 The University of North Carolina Press
All rights reserved
Set in Merope Basic by Westchester Publishing Services
Manufactured in the United States of America

Library of Congress Cataloging-in-Publication Data
Names: Batza, Katie author
Title: AIDS in the heartland : how unlikely coalitions created a blueprint for
   LGBTQ politics / Katie Batza.
Description: Chapel Hill : The University of North Carolina Press, [2025] |
   Includes bibliographical references and index.
Identifiers: LCCN 2025013910 | ISBN 9781469690483 cloth | ISBN 9781469690490
   paperback | ISBN 9781469690506 epub | ISBN 9781469690513 pdf
Subjects: LCSH: AIDS (Disease)—Political aspects—Middle West—History—
   20th century | LGBT activism—Middle West—History—20th century |
   BISAC: SOCIAL SCIENCE / Gender Studies | POLITICAL SCIENCE /
   Public Policy / Health Care
Classification: LCC RA643.84.M9 B3 2025 | DDC 362.19697/9200977—
   dc23/eng/20250621
LC record available at https://lccn.loc.gov/2025013910

Cover art: Aerial view of Earth. Oil painting by VikramRaghuvanshi /
iStock.com via Getty Images.

For product safety concerns under the European Union's General Product
Safety Regulation (EU GPSR), please contact gpsr@mare-nostrum.co.uk
or write to the University of North Carolina Press and Mare Nostrum
Group B.V., Mauritskade 21D, 1091 GC Amsterdam, The Netherlands.

To my constellation of family, born and chosen, that guide me, light my path, and encourage me to always wonder, and especially to the brightest among them, Kellie and Elliot. Also, Maya the Moose, wacky Watson, and Charlie, the very best dogs ever.

Contents

List of Illustrations ix

Introduction 1

CHAPTER ONE
The Heartland Imagined, Deployed, Erased, and Infected 9

CHAPTER TWO
Trouble at Home 29

CHAPTER THREE
Religion 52
The Politics of Piety

CHAPTER FOUR
Medicine from the Ground Up 78

CHAPTER FIVE
Political Posturing 102

Conclusion 122
Expanding Outward

Acknowledgments 133
Notes 137
Bibliography 153
Index 163

Illustrations

1.1 *Deep Creek Road, Flint Hills, KS* 10

1.2 *Terraced Plowing with Grass Waterway, April 1991* 11

1.3 *Fent's Prairie, Salina, Kansas, 1978* 13

1.4 *Footloose* 14

1.5 *Official Kansas Day Postcard* 16

3.1 *Praying Hands Monument, Graveyard, Route 54, Wichita, 1976* 53

4.1 *Repurposed Billboard West of Salina, Kansas, along I-70 7/13/2014 — 1:40 P.M.* 79

4.2 *Cemetery, February 1991* 100

5.1 *Empty Train Cars in Wheat Field near Friend, Kansas, May 2012* 103

C.1 *Fent's Prairie, Salina, Kansas, 1978* 127

AIDS in the Heartland

Introduction

Today, when I ask students to tell me about what the HIV/AIDS epidemic means to them, I get answers that differ in the extreme from the history I study. The young adults in my classrooms understand HIV/AIDS to be a historically serious illness, but one that is now treatable and even undetectable, given access to the proper medication, which many of my students often assume is accessible to everyone. The further in time we get from the early epidemic, the more HIV/AIDS seems to resemble smallpox or polio in their collective imaginations: an epidemiological event that has little impact on their day-to-day lives today. Their understanding of the HIV/AIDS epidemic flirts with apoliticism in a way that is unnerving and disturbing but ultimately gives me a greater commitment to the work of teaching the epidemic. Teaching the history of the epidemic feels increasingly like lifting a veil to reveal a gruesome past that diverges starkly from the simple expectation that the sick are tended to by caring medical professionals in white coats. The early HIV/AIDS epidemic is a lot of things, but attentive, white-coated care providers compassionately caring for the inexplicably ill do not resonate deeply with the history I know and the experiences of those who lived and died in those early decades.

Though the epidemic existed years before it was acknowledged, the MMWR reports of the summer of 1981 that marked the official beginning of the epidemic provide a strong jumping-off point to explore the social and political dimensions of HIV/AIDS. The very first line of the first-ever report of what would become AIDS began, "In the period October 1980–May 1981, 5 young men, all active homosexuals. . . ."[1] As the illness was immediately tied to homosexuals and then quickly to Black folks and intravenous drug users, the early demographic realities and reporting of the epidemic poured fuel on a smoldering culture war that took full form in the late 1960s, matured in the 1970s, and found itself at a crossroads at the start of the 1980s. The AIDS epidemic became a front line of the culture war of the 1980s that pitted political, fiscal, and social conservatives against nearly everyone else, especially homosexuals, people in poverty, and people of color. With the rise of the Religious Right and the increasing emphasis on neoliberalism that proclaimed personal responsibility and hard work as the solutions to all social ailments, the morality-infused and punitive response to any group in need of an organized state response set the stage for (several) calamitous crises that would have generational impacts on specific communities. Consider the full-throated war on drugs that had started a decade before, the rise of mass incarceration, the blaming of community poverty on personal shortcomings and blurred gender roles, the dwindling of the labor movement, and the state-echoed religious attacks on single mothers, homosexuals, and divorce. I often tell my students that HIV, like any virus, finds the optimal environment in which to thrive, but HIV went above and beyond, exploiting the normal epidemiological conditions like modes of transmission or resistance to or evasion of existing medications. If someone had concocted a recipe for a pandemic, there could not have been a better political moment or country for HIV to emerge in than the 1980s United States.

Against this political backdrop, HIV/AIDS quickly became a tool to vilify homosexuals, people of color, individuals experiencing poverty, and people who use substances, and to spur on American exceptionalism, particularly in relation to Africa and the Caribbean. As a result, those with HIV/AIDS in the early years of the epidemic rarely played the role of sick patients cared for by the doctors in the white coats. Instead, those with HIV/AIDS and their friends became activists, problem solvers, fighters, and deflectors of inhumane treatment within medical settings and beyond. The scene of the doctor attending at bedside was replaced by images of untouched hospital meal trays left outside the rooms of patients too weak to retrieve them, of rejection from existing care facilities to such an extent that local bars, convents, and community centers became makeshift hospice centers, and of community members standing in for professionals with medical training to provide care and love. Of course, this warped scene slowly shifted more toward the more standard doctors in white coats by the bedside, but only after much fighting, medical research, and lives lost. The history of AIDS is not set in a hospital or a research lab; instead, it is in the streets, in prisons, in bathhouses and gay bars, in the stories of friendships and love, and in the world HIV/AIDS activists created, even as many of them had a criminally shortened time in which to build it. It is not a medical history; it is a political one. It is a tragedy but also a story of resilience and power. It is a history, histories, that need telling and learning.

This book takes up that call, focusing on a region often excluded, detrimentally, from the HIV/AIDS history. However, *AIDS in the Heartland* goes beyond simply uncovering the history of the epidemic in this overlooked region—it also illuminates political forces and theoretical framings that not only shaped the AIDS response regionally and nationally in the early years of the epidemic but also continue to inform our world today, far beyond AIDS. AIDS in the American heartland has several distinct qualities that translate into both advantages and disadvantages for its study. First, the epidemic's spread pattern, hitting New York, San Francisco, and Los Angeles first, meant that the region benefited from extra time and opportunity to prepare, which the coastal cities did not have. Second, the density of the populations, particularly those subpopulations disproportionately infected by AIDS, meant that the AIDS epidemic had a vastly different scope in the Midwest than on the coasts. Third, the size of the affected populations informed the scope of AIDS activism and possible activism. LGBTQ communities across the Midwest were smaller, "not . . . as organized," and "not as vocal nor as open as their counterparts on the coasts," rendering some of the East Coast tactics unfeasible or meaningless in the Midwest context.[2] Finally, the local political landscape in the Midwest was, on average, much more conservative and reserved than those on the coasts.

The epidemic and the resulting activist response in the region illustrate an often less adversarial type of politics than associated with the coasts, but equally complex. In this way, *AIDS in the Heartland* takes an approach somewhat similar to Beth Bailey's important *Sex in the Heartland*, which explored the sexual liberation of the 1960s and 1970s in the small town of Lawrence, Kansas (where I write this book). Bailey finds that unlike the urban bohemian counterculture, gay liberation movements, and the hippie free love movement, the sexual liberation movement of the 1960s and 1970s grew from more nuanced and negotiated shifts in sexual culture and norms in small towns and less metropolitan settings.[3] Similarly, *AIDS in the Heartland* draws the responses to the AIDS epidemic of the 1980s and early 1990s away from the work of coastal chapters of ACT UP (though they were undoubtedly important) to explore how smaller communities responded to the epidemic. Without the urban political landscape and health infrastructure, lacking extensive gay political networks, and deeply enmeshed in the politics of self-sufficiency and neoliberalism, small towns and rural responses to AIDS offer a very different history, one that is equally important and impactful in our current politics. It is this quieter history that *AIDS in the Heartland* unearths and reveals as an important bedrock in the history of the epidemic.

The AIDS communities in the heartland were incredibly diverse in terms of sexuality, location within the region, race, income, religion, and role in the pandemic. I want to be clear that the demographics of those infected overwhelmingly skew toward queer people of all races and communities of color of all sexualities. However, the broader community of those who took up the AIDS response both included the infected and expanded far beyond them. Here again, scale was a significant factor, in that many who would have operated only on the peripheries (if at all) of the AIDS responses in coastal urban areas played more central roles in the heartland, often by coordinating multiple aspects of the response from housing and food to palliative care. For example, the cast of important characters in the heartland AIDS response extends to include crop duster pilots, church van drivers, convent heads, tribal leaders, and synagogue ladies, none of whom had HIV, and many of whom did not have HIV-positive people in their own families. However, the community of and for those impacted by HIV/AIDS was important to many people, not just those infected with the disease.

It was this broader constellation of AIDS responders in the region that ultimately became the topic of this book. When I moved to the region in 2014 to start my job at the University of Kansas, I assumed, based in part on the historiography I knew, that AIDS history and activism would not be a relatable or resonant discussion topic for my new neighbors and colleagues. Yet, surprisingly, colleagues, neighbors, strangers, wait staff at restaurants, mail carriers, fellow parents at the elementary school carnival, my realtor, and the sanitation worker who picked up my garbage—seemingly, almost everyone I interacted with—had a personal story about HIV/AIDS activism or caregiving just beneath the surface of introductory pleasantries. Perhaps the same was true when I lived in big cities on the coast, and I just didn't get to know everyone as much as I do in this small town I now call home. When my fellow heartlanders learned that my research at the time explored LGBTQ health infrastructure building and politics before AIDS, almost without fail, the conversation would turn to a discussion of a relative, friend, colleague, fellow parishioner, or acquaintance who either had HIV/AIDS, helped people with HIV/AIDS, attended funerals, or worked or volunteered for some HIV/AIDS-related service organization. Even if I had been in a major city on one of the coasts, it would have been unsettling how many people had connections to HIV/AIDS history. But I was in Kansas—Lawrence, Kansas, a blue dot of 90,000–115,000 people, depending on whether the university is in session. I was surprised, to say the least. Then, I began the search for archives and was astounded by the mostly untouched and vast offerings surrounding me.

Archives and interviews revealed that those in the HIV/AIDS community often operated at the peripheries of their other identity-based communities. For example, city public health workers saw Erise Williams as a strong potential AIDS activist and advocate in the Black community because he was always on the dance floor at the club.[4] Daniel Flier was a local drag performer and hairstylist who was willing to make some waves with his AIDS education–filled performances.[5] Sister Joann used her role in a Wichita convent to find hospice care and housing for people with HIV/AIDS.[6] Working within the HIV/AIDS community allowed members to center the disease and work in some of the more diverse coalitions in the region. Creating a home—through community, services, comradery, physical structures like housing units, or just a sense of healing, welcomeness, and belonging for people infected with and impacted by the disease—inspired much of the activism and activists of the region. After all, for many, the heartland was a place where HIV/AIDS community members were largely excluded or erased, a place deemed so unwelcoming that they had left, returning only under duress. AIDS responses in the region created new relationships to home through new communities.

However, this community was not free from structural racism, homophobia, classism, or norms of religious morality. After moving to the area from DC, one activist noticed that "people were more religious. . . . They were also more politically conservative in general. . . . The medicine is more conservative. . . . It was also very much racially divided."[7] This book explores the way that the scale of the region impacted the political tactics typically utilized by successful heartland HIV/AIDS organizers; generally, the need for compromise and widespread palatability had a moderating effect. Palatability and respectability became equally important, excluding HIV/AIDS community members in ways that regularly privileged whiteness, wealth, and conformity to gender norms. Home, even in the diverse community of people impacted by HIV/AIDS who either came to or stayed in the region, proved to be constantly in negotiation, fluid, and porous.

AIDS in the Heartland

AIDS in the Heartland unpacks the heartland as a site of diversity, resilience, innovation, political creativity, and widely influential strategies and historical lessons. As a whole, the book argues that the centering of respectability, home, and religion that proved salient in navigating the AIDS crisis in this region ultimately shaped the national framing of HIV/AIDS and the larger LGBTQ political agenda.[8] This work centers those most excluded from and harmed by both the heartland imaginary and the existing AIDS imaginary/historical literature—namely, queer folks and people of color and those who lived at the intersection of these identities. However, this is also a regional history, and uncovering the experiences of those most impacted by

HIV/AIDS requires a simultaneous deep exploration of whiteness, religious values, and neoliberal politics and structures.

The book is broken into five main thematic chapters, with the boundaries of each theme blurring into others, much like the geographic boundaries of the heartland. The first chapter, "The Heartland Imagined, Deployed, Erased, and Infected," lays out both the discursive and material landscapes on which this book rests. The heartland emerges as a vaguely defined geographic region with clear discursive boundaries that evoke a white, neoliberal, Christian politics frequently honed and deployed in the 1980s in the national political arena and mainstream media. With the concept of the heartland formed and functioning, the concepts of home and belonging ground the second chapter, "Trouble at Home." Home is a pliable and elusive concept that has proven theoretically lush in numerous intersecting academic fields. Chapter 2 paints a broad picture of home as a theoretical tool at work both in scholarship and in lived experiences in the heartland. While arguing that HIV/AIDS renders those it touches in the heartland "homeless," if not unhoused, this chapter also chronicles the arrival and scale of AIDS in the heartland and how AIDS bound some who had hoped to leave the region, pulled others who had left and become infected to return, and pushed others to move to the coasts where they felt more useful in fighting AIDS's impact. It defines the idiosyncrasies of the heartland epidemic while also illuminating the complex articulations of "home" as a deeply contested place of departure, reckoning, nurturing, and family that molded the AIDS experience there.

Chapter 3, "Religion: The Politics of Piety," builds on these notions of home to explore a key animating force in the heartland AIDS response: religion. Religion was the backbone not only for bigotry, epitomized perhaps most notoriously by Fred Phelps, but also, and perhaps more surprisingly, for a compassionate and well-established social service response to the HIV/AIDS epidemic. The type of religious response was often directly related to the deployment of respectability politics and the emphasis placed on homosexuality, which in turn was deeply tied to materializations of home. Religion appears as the driving force behind this posturing in myriad ways explored in this chapter.

Chapter 4, "Medicine from the Ground Up," examines the scientific and medical innovations created and deployed in the region. Faced with a relative dearth of medical research institutions and patients spread across vast landscapes, scientists and medical providers faced challenges unfathomable to their coastal counterparts. A small handful of medical professionals found themselves going far beyond the role of typical medical care provider and into the worlds of fundraising, community organizing, public speaking, legislation, and state sex education development and rollout. In these medical trailblazers, the power of respectability, the heartland imaginary, and the neoliberal notion of bootstrapping emerge again as critical forces propelling the regional AIDS response.

While the entire history of the HIV/AIDS response in the heartland is a political tale, "Political Posturing," the fifth chapter, unearths the emergence of heartland AIDS-related political organizations specifically. There is a surprising diversity of the political footings on which activists built these organizations. As religious-based efforts sought to bridge racial divisions, the purely political realm allowed more space for Black-specific and "color-blind" (predominantly white) organizations. Meanwhile, Native communities also found unique organizations and ways to shine a light on the idiosyncratic failures and historical legacy of the Indian Health Service. However, the most successful (in terms of longevity and financial solvency) of the political organizations born of the heartland AIDS crisis were religiously adjacent and deployed ideals of respectability and neoliberalism that centered individuality, privacy, and self-sufficiency, showcasing how this region's realities conflict with the national historical AIDS narrative. Importantly, a closer look at these organizations also shows that they were built to work in tandem with more politically unpalatable organizations to maximize the response to the needs of people with HIV/AIDS.

The conclusion, "Expanding Outward," traces the white imaginary into today, exposing the continued impacts of the heartland AIDS response and the political tactics and systems it engaged. It builds to examine how the region's AIDS response inspired the national LGBT political platform in the 1990s and 2000s to center palatable AIDS-adjacent topics like marriage and military service—so much so that Iowa became the first state to adopt marriage equality. This recasts the heartland as having significantly informed, if not driven, the LGBT political agenda in the late twentieth and early twenty-first centuries.

CHAPTER ONE

The Heartland Imagined, Deployed, Erased, and Infected

> It is not easy to see things in the middle, rather than looking down on them from above or up at them from below, or from left to right or from right to left: try it, you'll see that everything changes.
> —GILLES DELEUZE AND FÉLIX GUATTARI, *A Thousand Plateaus*

"The heartland" is an ambiguous shorthand for an area smaller than "flyover country" (another amorphous concept) but still decidedly in the country's center, somewhere. Many scholars and residents alike have tried to clarify the exact boundaries of the heartland, only to be confounded by places like East St. Louis, Illinois, Kansas City, Kansas, or Cedar Bluffs, Iowa, which straddle state borders with blatant disregard for a scholar's need for legibility in describing the geography to larger audiences, most of whom have never been to the heartland, let alone its contested peripheries.[1] Depending on the scholar or resident, the heartland can overlap with states as far-flung as Ohio and Oklahoma, or North Dakota and Arkansas, or Indiana and Montana. Vast, state-sized topographies of flat agricultural scenes come to mind, though in actuality, these have much more movement and elevation than assumed. Proximity to rurality combined with the absence of an ocean boundary seems to be a nearly universal defining feature of the heartland, as does a widespread political and religious conservatism with notable liberal towns, or "blue dots." As a scholar of HIV/AIDS, I see that another useful way to visualize the heartland is by imagining a photographic negative of areas historians have thus far explored as important to HIV/AIDS history.

I am less concerned with the exact boundaries of the heartland and even what binds it together as a region. Rather than cartography, the ambiguity and the contrast of the heartland as a place and concept are critical to this research.[2] I am more concerned with the heartland as a discursive or theoretical space than as a material or physical space. While we may argue over where the heartland is, we all agree it isn't on the Eastern Seaboard or the West Coast. It is not New York City or San Francisco. I find this term perfect for exactly what this book seeks to explore. In this study, the amorphous heartland (that area so often excluded from HIV/AIDS history) is the focal point.

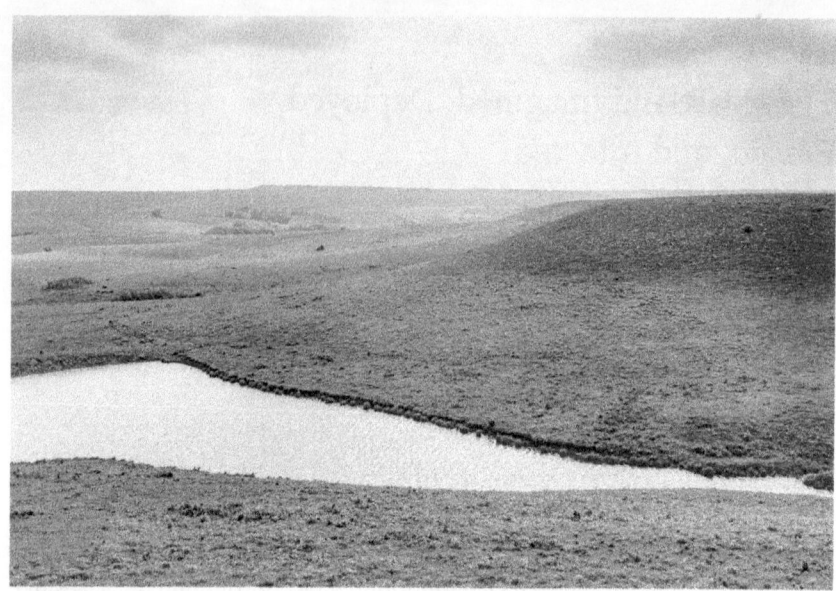

FIGURE 1.1 Earl Iversen, *Deep Creek Road, Flint Hills, KS*, 1979. Gelatin silver print. Spencer Museum of Art, University of Kansas, Gift of the artist, 1981.0063.

As we center our attention on the heartland, it appears at the heart of the country—not just the geographic center, but the heart in its many metaphorical senses—doing the work of circulating ideas, nutrients, and action to the extremities; as the metaphorical bodily site for care and love; as the place idealized and longed for in times of danger or sickness. Despite the expectations for a one-dimensional narrative from a one-dimensional region (as the existing literature and narratives might inspire), this history reveals a multilayered, diverse landscape. Landscape photography illustrates this point. The expected heartland landscape reveals the often hazy, romanticized image of virgin land with endless horizons that is often associated with the region, which at once orients and disorients as distances and details are hard to see. Earl Iversen's photograph *Deep Creek Road*, for example, shows a clear, exact location, but that location communicates nowhere specific (see figure 1.1). These romanticized versions of photography resonate with the notion of the heartland imaginary as both somewhere and nowhere, as both clearly defined and largely inferred, and as both inhabited (how else would it be photographed?) and virgin.

Another photographer, Terry Evans, takes a decidedly different tack that I hope to also employ in this research. She explores the heartland from two vantage points: from the air (aerial photography) and from the perspective

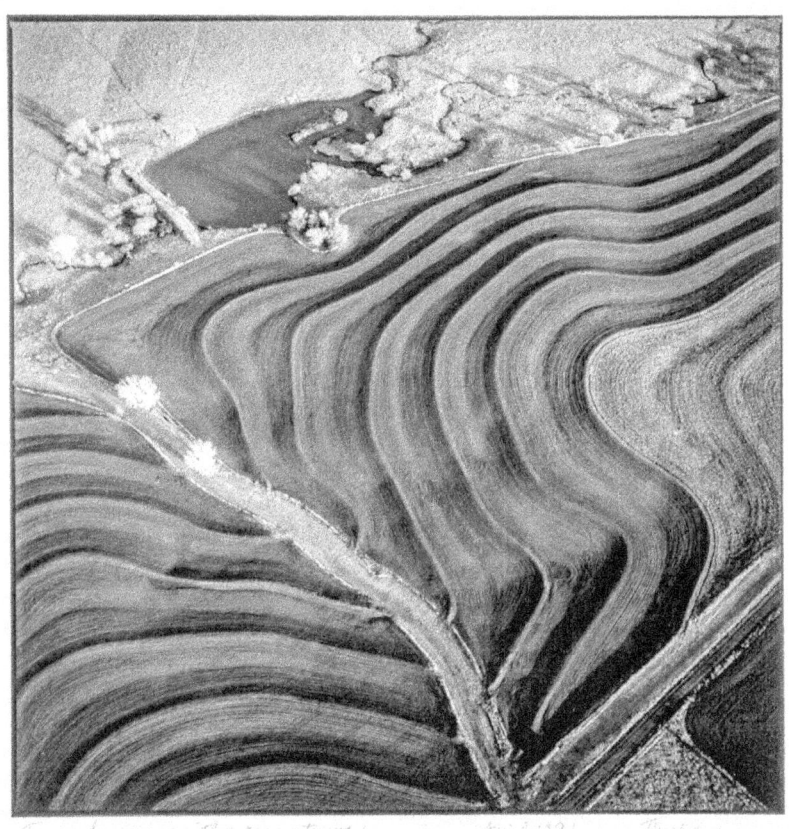

FIGURE 1.2 Terry Evans, *Terraced Plowing with Grass Waterway, April 1991*. Gelatin silver print. Spencer Museum of Art, University of Kansas, Museum purchase: Helen Foresman Spencer Art Acquisition Fund, 1992.0033.

of looking straight down from a standing position. In looking at the heartland (both as a concept and a landscape) from these angles, we see much greater complexity. Rather than looking out, the act of searching within the landscape proves much more illuminating about the place and its complexities. From directly above, a field reveals a carefully molded cartography of thoughtful formations to shape a certain kind of growth, with carefully planned shade spots, manipulation of water, and the grooves and tracks left by farming machinery. In short, these new angles remove much of the romantic virginity of rural landscapes depicted in images that look out toward a horizon to reveal the labor, planning, and interlocking systems on which farming relies (see figure 1.2).

Far from untouched and natural, this landscape is filled with carefully crafted nuance and symbiosis. The current AIDS historiography either fails to explore the heartland or does so with a horizontal view in which much of the labor and intricacy is lost. This more nuanced depiction of the land evokes another story that embraces the region as a pivotal character: *The Wizard of Oz*. Like this famous 1939 film, an adaptation of L. Frank Baum's 1900 children's fantasy novel *The Wonderful Wizard of Oz*, the history of HIV/AIDS in the heartland, presented here from a more aerial vantage point, is a political allegory filled with a violent and unfamiliar beginning, unlikely collaborators, bizarre and frightening dangers, cross-regional migrations, and a quest for home.[3]

A growing number of queer and straight scholars and theorists have turned to the heartland or the middle of the country to undertake a wide variety of productive theorizing and scholarship. Works by Scott Herring, J. Halberstam, Colin Johnson, Siobahn Somerville, Toni Morrison, Ryan Cartwright, Doris Davenport, and Beth Clement, and, more broadly, studies on trans theory represent just a smattering of the scholarship that has found fertile ground in the heartland topography and history to pick apart a variety of hegemonic binaries that inflict harm on marginalized bodies and histories by reinforcing racism, transphobia, homophobia, and xenophobia through erasure. In one vein, this work has identified heartland histories that include queer folks and people of color as rural residents, disrupting the imaginary whiteness of the region. In another vein, scholars have used the region as a sort of theoretical simile—an example of queer time and space for J. Halberstam, an "in-between" space, as Marquis Bey might say, or a site of enmeshment in the terms of Sara Ahmed.[4] The wide-open spaces of this region are largely unexplored by scholars but they brim with possibility as they overflow with contradictions, nuance, isolation, interdependence, and so much more. We are now finding that the heartland, too long rendered as boring or empty, sparks the imagination in exciting ways for scholars across many fields that disrupt our larger understandings. *AIDS in the Heartland* joins in this usage of the heartland as both an actual place and theoretical playground to dislodge and discern hegemonic structures at play in existing AIDS histories. The heartland is a place to revel in the knots and tangles, the unexpected connections and site of interreliance, the cycle of life, which Terry Evans captures so well simply by looking down (see figure 1.3).

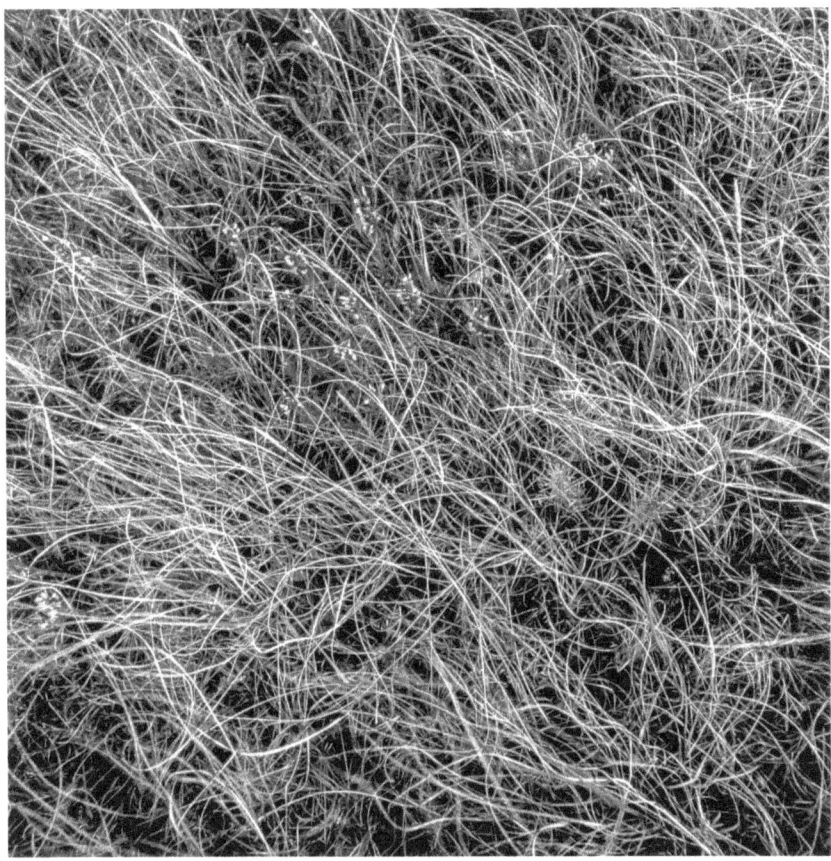

FIGURE 1.3 Terry Evans, *Fent's Prairie, Salina, Kansas, 1978*. Spencer Museum of Art, University of Kansas, Gift of Terry Evans, 1980.0147.

The White Heartland Imaginary

In the 1980s, the nebulous heartland served as an ideological home for much of white America "as a geographic entity and as a discursive formation."[5] If, as B. J. Schulman and many others have argued, the 1970s saw the southernization of the nation, I would argue that the 1980s saw the rise of the heartland in a similar vein.[6] In fact, the heartland provides an incredibly important form of whiteness that isn't Southern and that came to dominate in the 1980s and 1990s. This non-Southern whiteness allows for a greater distance between whiteness and overt and violent racism. Much of this formation relied on the willful erasure of the history of the heartland as a place of

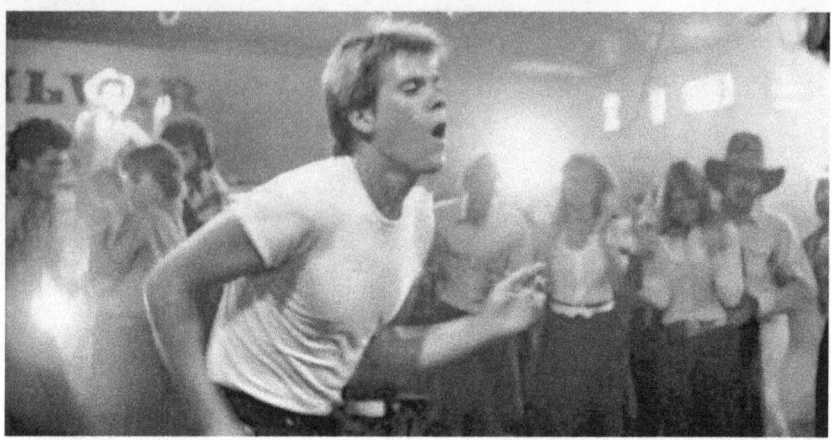

FIGURE 1.4 Still from *Footloose*, Paramount Pictures, 1984.

stolen land, forced migrations, and harmful farming practices. It also leaned heavily on Christianity, heterosexuality, and conservative politics, which, in many ways, became synonymous with the idealized depiction of the region.

Popular culture did much of this work. For example, the 1989 film *Field of Dreams* had Kevin Costner infusing the collective imaginary with the possibility of Iowa farm fields. The heartland became the backdrop for an imagined ideal for white America, a sort of shared innocence and experience, where the perceived overwhelming whiteness of the population allowed for a false sense of immunity from the Black and white racial upheavals of the postwar period and the violence of slavery and segregation. The existence of Indian reservations and Native nations at once removed from white view and deferred accountability for the lands stolen and soaked with violence and injustice for this white imaginary ideological home. Rather, under the guise of this heartland ideal, rebellion and struggle took the much more palatable form of Kevin Bacon in the 1984 film *Footloose* fighting for the right to have a high school dance (see figure 1.4).[7]

Bacon's character does significant work to expose the boundaries of the white heartland imaginary as he carefully weaves together the role of the white outsider with a dedication to hard labor (working and dancing in a granary), determined heterosexuality while secretly giving dancing lessons to a cowboy boots–wearing heartland boy, and deferral, if not devotion, to the religious standards of his new home. In the end, he perseveres to win a night of wholesome fun. The subtext is clear: it is his whiteness, straightness, ability to speak the language of religion and conservatism, and hard work that allow him to successfully navigate the outsider status in the heartland.

Success would surely not be so assured if Bacon's character had been Black, queer, rich, perceived as lazy, or non-Christian. In this way, even in its depiction of an outsider in the heartland, *Footloose* helps craft and reinforce the white heartland imaginary.

Of course, popular culture wasn't alone in the crafting of the white heartland imaginary. The heartland was and is a political tool occasionally called on to do the work of idealizing and convincing a larger audience to act a certain way, often against their own best interests.[8] Colonization, westward expansion, and Manifest Destiny necessitated the forging of this particular tool by politicians and wealthy capitalists to lure colonizers from the East Coast to partake in a romanticized world-building, despite the fact that for those who did so, their life expectancies often dropped significantly and their survival and lived experiences were much more laborious.

A postcard from 1911 (figure 1.5) evokes this early version of the heartland white imaginary. Here, three important themes emerge. First, Kansas is a place of order where the hay bales and oil wells are evenly spaced, and even the arrangement of the cows seems symmetrical. Second, Kansas is a place of movement, work, and technology, attested by the factory and trains in the distance, not to mention the automobile on the road. Third, Kansas is white. The white woman with the toga is the only person large enough that her race can be discerned, but swaddled in a Roman toga and holding a mirror out to the viewer of the postcard, she embodies the postcard's efforts to erase the existence of Native people while simultaneously beckoning the presumably white viewer to imagine themselves there. Thus, the postcard presents Kansas as a place of order, hard work, and whiteness, with each of these components interlocking with the others.

In this earlier incarnation, the heartland imaginary was carefully crafted around the outcomes desired by national political and business leaders to align a narrative of a romantic, self-sacrificing work ethic of middle- and working-class whites (not to mention the work of racial warfare) with patriotism and particular brands of freedom and liberty. As a result, large swaths of the mostly white electorate moved westward, building infrastructure, invading and colonizing Native spaces, and all the while, granting more power to political leaders and industry titans by expanding their empires and coffers.

The 1980s saw a similar use of the white heartland imaginary as a political and rhetorical tool by government and business but also replaced the common culprit of injustice and inequality from the class warfare of the early and mid-twentieth century with the villain of liberalism. What better tool to deploy than a region whose identity is tightly bound to self-sufficiency, hard

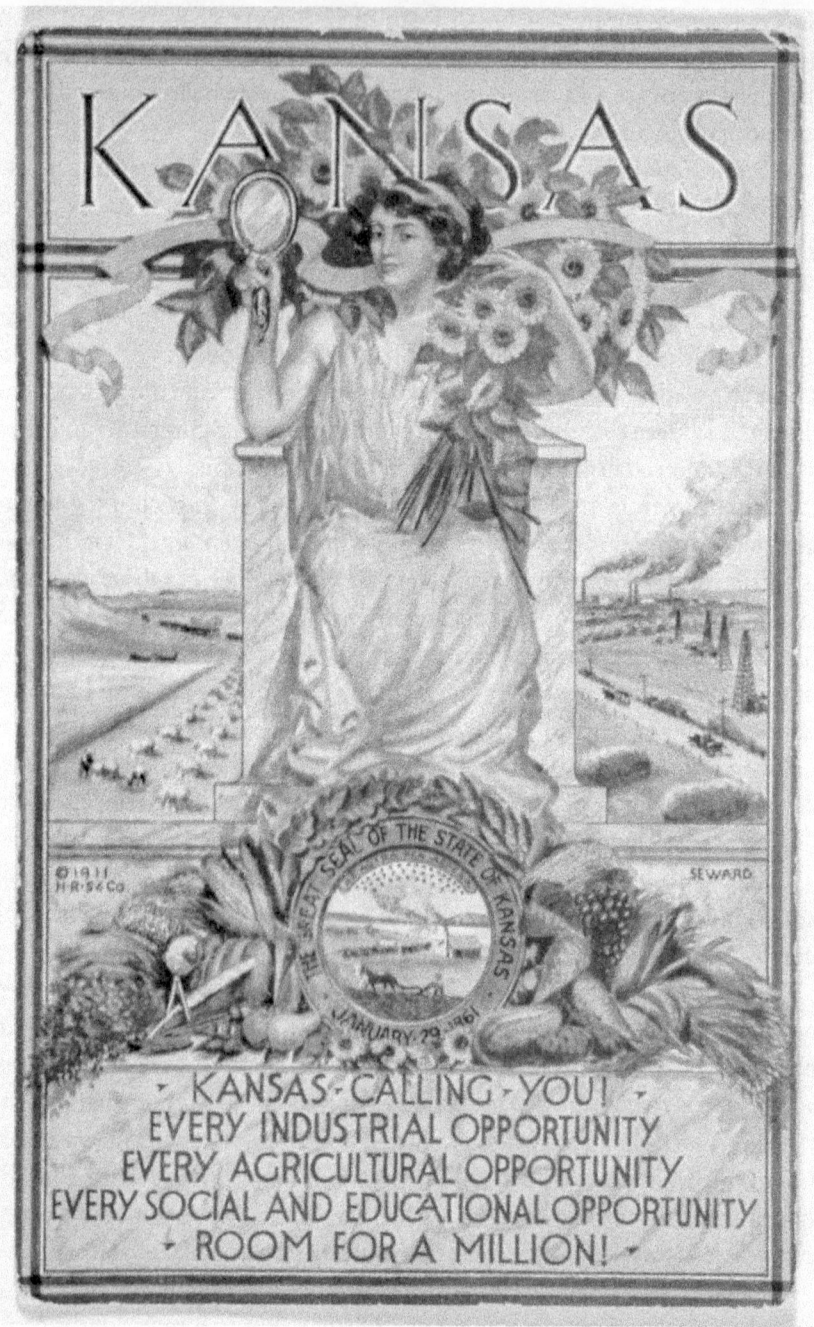

FIGURE 1.5 Coy Avon Seward, *Official Kansas Day Postcard*, 1911. Offset color lithograph. Spencer Museum of Art, University of Kansas, gift in memory of Mildred Seward Pierce, 2006.0176.

labor, whiteness, and Christianity to legitimize and excite the electorate to embrace a politics that eviscerated social safety nets, weakened workers' rights, revolutionized structural racism, and nurtured the rise of the Religious Right? Thomas Frank's book *What's the Matter with Kansas? How Conservatives Won the Heart of America* (2004) chronicles the rise of a populist and anti-elitist conservatism in Kansas despite its rich history as a site of progressivism, labor struggle, and abolition.[9] While his work focuses more on the electoral politics and policies of Kansas, the white heartland imaginary refers to the larger ethos that both allowed for these politics and policies and was born from them. It also expands far beyond the boundaries of the state of Kansas. The heartland personifies an economic and political ideology that made invisible the role of the state and capitalism in creating disparities, and instead laid blame squarely at the feet of those who did not fit into the white heartland imaginary for various reasons.[10]

With respect to the AIDS response in the region, the white heartland imaginary's most important components are the wholesale erasure of class division and all negative effects of capitalism, the insistence on neoliberalism (by which I mean the transfer of responsibilities formally held by the state onto the individual citizen), and the creation of a form of national whiteness beyond the South. Through the lens of the white heartland imaginary, the vast swath of people living in the United States became de facto middle class (from corporate executives to farmers and from factory workers to bankers), simultaneously capable of caring for their own needs and bound together by the white heartland imaginary culture. When AIDS rendered poor many of the infected and created communities unable to handle the scope of needs related to the epidemic, the construct of the white heartland imaginary allowed for these realities to be seen as personal failings rather than failings of the State or society, and the natural consequence of bucking the culture. Furthermore, as AIDS began to disproportionately hit communities of color, the white heartland imaginary provided a deflection of the racism embedded in the villainization and dismissal of these groups, because racism in the heartland "didn't exist" when compared to the overt and violent racism of the desegregating South of the previous decades. Of course, these components of the white heartland imaginary played out simultaneously with other tools designed to render those infected homeless, both discursively and materially. Namely, mass incarceration, the criminalization of HIV/AIDS, and a new articulation of what Steven Thrasher dubs "the viral underclass" in his book by the same name worked in tandem with the larger concept of the white heartland imaginary to "make safe" those who belonged in the white heartland imaginary and punish those who did not.[11] For those with HIV/AIDS, "home" became increasingly precarious, under attack, and denied as they were marked as outsiders by the infection itself, let alone the intersectional markers of outsider status like homosexuality, nonwhiteness, and poverty.

When the early 1980s saw family farmers grapple with increased inflation, decreased property values, and diminishing market prices, the region also became an example of idealized white bootstrapping and "grit," which propped up neoliberal economic and social welfare policies across the country.[12] Bruce Springsteen, though from New Jersey, tapped into this shared white identity of grit, struggle, and a sense of beautiful desolation in the heartland imaginary with his 1982 album *Nebraska*. The region became synonymous with an imaginary white American working- and middle-class ideal that valorized struggle, perseverance, and independence. White heartland residents embraced this image to such an extent that the region overwhelmingly voted to give Ronald Reagan a second presidential term in 1984, despite the economic pain many had endured under his leadership.[13] In short, the region's imagined features created the silhouette of the ideal American citizen: white, hardworking, religious, straight, family oriented, and socially conservative—the venerated and idolized pioneer, weathered by the devastating dustbowl, matured by the 1980s.

The Heartland Reality

The heartland's imaginary relationship to historical violence is an important piece of the discursive formation of the region. The imagined heartland history allows for nearly complete white avoidance of racialized violence or politics and requires historical slippage to paint this picture. In her essay "Home," Toni Morrison addresses this conundrum with her usual eloquence: "It is difficult to sign race while designing racelessness." She also explains, "I have never lived, nor has any of us, in a world in which race did not matter."[14] Navigating a racially innocuous history requires the imaginary heartland to do a bit of time traveling and tap dancing in relation to Native nations and peoples. The frontier battles with Native people were a defining feature of the imagined toughness of white pioneers. But the white innocence on which the heartland imaginary relies comes from a different time altogether: after the forced relocations of Native people. Once they were "settled" on the (white) imagined "sanctuaries" of reservations, the heartland was once again presented as racially neutral, available for white dominance and ubiquity without the messiness of historical racial accountability or reckoning. Here, the heartland imaginary dismisses nonwhite actors to the regional and historical wings, allowing for an overwhelming whiteness to stand in for the region. Meanwhile, life on the reservations is often defined by poverty, poor resources and infrastructure, and limited employment opportunities.

Though the question of expanding slavery in the region ultimately ignited the Civil War, the heartland is often portrayed as largely tangential to not just the war but also the systemic racial violence, including slavery, that both instigated the war and perpetuated afterward. Seen as the far-flung borderlands or the frontier during the early nineteenth century, the heartland is imagined as a racially neutral landscape between Black and white folk, where adventurous and hardworking white pioneers only occasionally interacted with non-Native people of color, thus allowing the imagined heartland to be unburdened by the stain of slavery (and the resulting social and political struggles) that marred the South and former British colonies.[15] The heartland imaginary simply ignores the possibility of Black folk in the region, both during the initial "settling" of the area and even much later as the Great Migration of the early twentieth century has Black migration terminating either "north" of the ambiguous heartland border or in the few cities within the region wherein urbanity allows for some deviation from the heartland imaginary ideal.[16]

The invisibility of Latinx and African migrants is the final piece of the imagined history of the heartland. By the 1980s, as the AIDS epidemic began to take shape, the heartland had experienced several waves of migration, particularly from Central and South America and Somalia.[17] With the growth of corporate farming practices in the region, migrants became an important fixture not just during crop harvest times but also, more importantly, in meatpacking plants across the region. Much of this work occurs in small towns in predominantly rural landscapes like Garden City, Kansas, and Grand Island, Nebraska, with proximity to farms and slaughterhouses but also far removed from the majority of meat consumers.[18] Thus, the production of the meat and those who do the labor of slaughter and packaging fall under the same veil of willful invisibility that shrouds the need for grappling with multiple forms of violence.

In reality, the heartland, like the rest of the country, is a cartography of racial violence, struggle, and resilience. The region is deeply entwined with Native peoples and cultures. Though the white imaginary has whitewashed the landscape as much as possible, the ground is soaked with the blood and tears of Native peoples violently evicted, marched across, and forced to relocate on this landscape. While the region is home to many of the existent reservations and the political and cultural hubs for a wide array of Native nations, it is also the backdrop of the Trail of Tears, former Indian boarding schools, and ongoing battles over sovereignty and violence, particularly against women.[19] This is geography on which Native people have maintained languages, cultures, and sovereignty against impossible odds and in the face of ruthlessly creative efforts to erase them from the land, from the protests at Standing Rock to the commemoration of the largest mass hanging in US history (thirty-eight Dakota tribe members in 1862, as part of the US-Dakota War), to the vibrant college campus of Haskell University celebrating Native histories and cultures.

Far from being devoid of Black folk during the Civil War era, the heartland has been the backdrop for enslavement and terror, both legally permitted in states like Missouri and Arkansas and in "free states" like Kansas, where proslavery forces violently raided towns, as in Quantrill's Raid in Lawrence, Kansas.[20] Beyond the period of legalized bondage, white violence against Black bodies in the region included intense segregation, lynching, redlining, voter intimidation, rioting, and the application of economic limitations, like in other parts of the country. There are countless examples to draw from, ranging from the widespread devastation of the Tulsa Race Massacre of 1921 to the lynching of three Black men in 1882 by a white mob in Lawrence, Kansas.[21] However, the region has also been home to sites of tremendous Black resilience and thriving. Nicodemus, Kansas, became the first Black community west of the Mississippi on its founding in 1877 by freed enslaved people from Kentucky, and it stands as the only remaining Western community established by Black Americans after the Civil War.[22] The heartland also offers a deep Black cultural tradition that includes writers like Langston Hughes and countless musicians such as Charlie Parker, as well as culinary gifts that define the region, like BBQ. Though the heartland imaginary is a stark shade of white, the heartland reality includes rich Black histories and communities.

Though the heartland imaginary feigns ignorance, the ground here has been fertilized with dreams for a better future and spoiled by exploitative labor practices and xenophobia against immigrants. The heartland's relationship with immigrants is deeply divided along racial lines. On the one hand, the region is dotted with small towns that still speak German, Swedish, Norwegian, Polish, or Dutch and celebrate those cultures. However, even these echoes of historical immigration have been folded into the imagined whiteness of the larger region. The Dust Bowl, an environmental disaster almost entirely made by white men, still lingers as a shared misery and as formative in the imagined white toughness of the area. On the other hand, as later immigrants arrived from Latin and South American countries rather than Europe, the existing second and third generations of white immigrants became a phalanx of whiteness that stood in contrast to Latinx folks, pushing them to the peripheries of towns and labor forces. Consequently, Latinx immigrants exist outside this venerated earlier migration, even as they have taken up much of the labor (but not the land or wealth) of farming, whether in the form of harvesting, slaughtering, or packaging agricultural bounty. Similarly, African (mostly Somali) immigrants have found work in meatpacking plants across the region but remain exposed to violence emanating from the white heartland imaginary.

The heartland reality requires acknowledgment of and grappling with not only the various violent histories of this landscape but also the violence of the present. The white heartland imaginary fuels the exclusion of people who challenge white heartland ideals while simultaneously emboldening those who embody the white heartland imaginary to police and enforce white heartland imaginary ideals. Inevitably, this leads to violence and hate crimes. In 1993, Brandon Teena, a transgender man, was raped and later murdered in Humboldt, Nebraska, by two white men. His story was later the inspiration for the 1999 film *Boys Don't Cry*. Just five years later, in 1998, three white men, two of whom were vocal white supremacists, murdered James Byrd Jr. by dragging his body behind a pickup truck for three miles, resulting in his decapitation. After driving for more than a mile more, they dumped Byrd's broken and dismembered body in front of a Black church. Also that year, a University of Wyoming student, Matthew Shepard, was beaten, tortured, and tied to a fencepost and left to die in Laramie, Wyoming, because he was gay. In 2016, an FBI raid thwarted a plot by three white militia members in Garden City, Kansas, to bomb an apartment complex housing mostly Somali and Muslim residents.[23] All of these violent and hate-fueled murders went on to inspire important pieces of hate crimes legislation, yet the crimes themselves were inspired, in part, by the white heartland imaginary. The violence continues even as the imaginary heartland remains a place "where nothing happens" and where whiteness is "free" from the stain of the racism of the South.

Erasure in the Heartland

The heartland as a discursive formation, as a white imaginary, is harmful not just because it ignores the historical and contemporary realities of many who live in the region but also because its act of ignoring and erasing makes the thriving of those who defy the white imaginary harder to imagine and to actualize.[24] The heartland imaginary is ever present in the history of HIV/AIDS in the region, either as an animating force or as an obstacle to work around. If queerness or racial diversity appears in the popular culture of the imagined heartland of the 1980s, it is often through the popular culture genre of horror or crime, as Scott Herring explores in his analysis of hixploitation films (a genre of exploitation film that negatively depicts rural whites).[25] Though these works technically acknowledge the existence of difference in the region, it is only to act out a corrective and often a violent backlash against it either through pathologizing or victimizing those portrayed as different, thus fortifying the discursive imaginary of homogenous whiteness, straightness, and religiosity. Another critical example of situating queerness in the white heartland imaginary appears in the form of an episode of *The Oprah Winfrey Show* in July 1987 titled "AIDS Comes to a Small Town." Winfrey centered the episode on the community response to Mike Sisco, a gay man infected with HIV, swimming in the town pool in Williamson, West Virginia. The town closed down the town pool, and news of the brief swim made headlines in the local newspaper the next day. Winfrey's approach gives voice to the pain and violence enacted on Sisco and his family while also portraying the small town as quintessentially heartland and insular. While more nuanced and sophisticated than a horror movie, the episode ultimately reinforces the white heartland imaginary ideals, made deeply apparent when one Williamson resident explains, "Mike had a choice. He shirked his responsibility as a man," suggesting not only that homosexuality is a choice but that heterosexuality is a responsibility of heartland ideals.[26] Meanwhile, although the episode successfully created greater compassion for Sisco on a national level, by highlighting this highly negative example it also clearly communicated that homosexuality and small towns do not mix well.

While queer theorists and historians have started to unpack the complexity of the region, the assumed homogeneity ascribed by the heartland imaginary has, in many ways, been unchallenged by the existing literature of the early AIDS epidemic. Existing depictions of the early AIDS epidemic, whether in academic writings, in popular culture, or in the public imaginary, are tied deeply to an urban, often coastal, geography or broad national narratives that overlook the heartland. Perhaps the most famous and widely read book about the epidemic in popular culture, *And the Band Played On*, did significant work to conflate the gay community with the coasts and largely ignored even the existence of the vast swaths of the country as it bounced from

New York to Los Angeles and from San Francisco to Atlanta.[27] Of course, cities had dense populations of communities disproportionately impacted by early HIV/AIDS, which in turn led to the bulk of national infections, deaths, and social services for the affected. While the works of scholars such as Tamar Carrol, Sarah Schulman, Darius Bost, Dan Royles, Cathy Cohen, Salonee Bhaman, Nic John Ramos, Jonathan Bell, Emily Hobson, and Jennifer Brier, among others, do tremendous work in uncovering important aspects of the history of AIDS, they remain firmly bound to the coasts or the few major cities that lie in between them.[28] While crucial to the growing historical study of HIV/AIDS, these depictions, taken together as a whole, ignore the nonurban, noncoastal experience to the extent of erasure. To be clear, none of these scholars intend to do the work of erasure—quite the opposite. However, the sum of the field ignores the heartland, particularly the rural/nonurban heartland. This coastal focus provides an incomplete understanding of HIV/AIDS and harms those impacted by HIV/AIDS who did not live in coastal urban landscapes. It renders vast swaths of the country not in coastal urban centers one-dimensional, oversimplified, and seemingly irrelevant. In short, the existing AIDS literature reifies the heartland imaginary. It also denies the reality of migration.

Ignoring the history of heartland people who grappled with HIV/AIDS in the 1980s and 1990s does the work of the heartland imaginary by painting over not only the experiences but also the existence of people of color, queer folks, and others who were impacted by HIV/AIDS who lived in the heartland. The consequence of this oversight has real effects on historians grappling with this history, but also (and more importantly) it impacts those who live in or want to live in the heartland, as it becomes harder to live there and imagine it matters.[29] In a way, the existing history is compounding the work of structural racism, homophobia, and centering of the urban in how it blunts our collective imaginary of the region as a site of possibility—of possible political creativity, of diversity, of coalition building, of widely applicable tactics and historical lessons.

Infecting the Heartland

The emergence of the HIV/AIDS epidemic in the heartland is vastly different from the coastal trajectories that early on inspired anxious pleas in the *New York Native* by soon-to-be AIDS activist Larry Kramer and cautionary handmade posters taped to pharmacy windows in San Francisco's Castro neighborhood warning of the impending calamity.[30] The commonly told, coastally focused history of HIV/AIDS "starts" in 1981 with a series of reports in both medical and mass media news outlets describing a new disease with a strange constellation of symptoms from skin lesions to an unusual form of pneumonia among homosexual men. The name "AIDS" emerged in 1983 after several discriminatory and inaccurate predecessors, including "gay cancer" and "gay-related immune deficiency." The discovery of HIV didn't occur until the following year, and a screening test became available a full year after that, in 1985. By then, more than 130,000 people had been diagnosed with HIV in the United States, and more than 30,000 had died. It was also in 1985 that then-president Ronald Reagan uttered the word "AIDS" publicly for the first time, after a long delay that indicated his willful ignorance of the epidemic that would, by the end of his second term, claim more lives in the United States than the number of US soldiers who died in the Vietnam War. In large part due to this failure in leadership, federal research funding for HIV/AIDS and services for the people suffering from it were anemic at best and nonexistent at worst.

In gay enclaves in major metropolitan areas, complex grassroots webs of care and services emerged, most famously the Gay Men's Health Crisis in New York, which became immediately overwhelmed by the sheer number of infected and scrambled to meet the needs of a quickly growing population of deeply stigmatized and very ill people. In addition to the deadliness of AIDS itself, violence and discrimination against people with HIV/AIDS and the larger gay community with which it was associated left many without housing, work, medical care, and community. The year 1987 marked a turning point in the epidemic in two ways: first, with the FDA (Food and Drug Administration) approval of AZT, the first (though often ineffective) medication approved to treat patients with HIV/AIDS; and second, with the founding of the radical activist organization ACT UP (AIDS Coalition to Unleash Power) in New York City. These activists took to the streets with disruptive and creative protests that eventually resulted in changes to FDA drug approval procedures, federal funding for HIV/AIDS, and efforts to educate the broader public. This group also battled the CDC (Centers for Disease Control) for two years to change the definition of HIV/AIDS to include more opportunistic infections, including gynecological infections. As a result, in 1993, many more women with HIV/AIDS gained access to treatments and services previously denied to them. By then, the epidemic had exploded far beyond the initial demographics initially associated with the disease, impacting women, children, and heterosexuals, particularly in communities of color. In 1996 researchers discovered a drug "cocktail," HAART, or highly active antiretroviral therapy, which effectively transformed HIV/AIDS from an automatic death sentence to a manageable chronic illness for those who could access and afford the treatment. Far from over, the epidemic up to that point had illuminated the apathy of the federal government and the herculean power of communities (particularly the LGBTQ communities) to help each other and effect change.

The differences between the coastal and heartland experiences of the arrival of HIV/AIDS come down to the timing of the disease, the number of cases, and density in terms of available resources and the spread of populations across a vast landscape. The AIDS epidemic in the heartland was both earlier and later in arriving as part of what we commonly think of as the burgeoning AIDS crisis of the 1980s. A Black sixteen-year-old St. Louis resident named Robert Rayford died on May 15, 1969, after a near-complete shutdown of his immune system that had befuddled doctors at City Hospital.[31] Though it took until 1985 for antibody tests to be run on long-stored tissue samples to clarify the cause of Rayford's passing, it is now widely believed to be the first known HIV/AIDS-related death in the United States.[32] We know very little about Rayford or how he contracted the virus. He was a low-income Black teen who had never traveled out of the region. He first presented in 1968 with swelling, fatigue, chlamydia, and a very low immune response. His death would reveal that he also had small lesions all over his body, a rare form of cancer nearly unprecedented among Black teenagers—Kaposi's sarcoma. His evasion of questions posed by doctors and nurses led some to presume he had cognitive disabilities and others to point to potential sexual abuse, neither of which can be substantiated. In any case, his history remains a mystery, as does the specific strain of HIV that killed him, because all remaining tissue samples were destroyed in the flood waters of Hurricane Katrina in 2005.[33] His case was the only one reported in the region for over a decade. Even as cases of what would become known as HIV/AIDS made their unwelcome appearance in the summer of 1981 as the CDC's *Morbidity and Mortality Weekly Report* (*MMWR*) noted unusual deaths among gay men in New York and Los Angeles, the heartland remained unscathed.[34] Iowa didn't report its first case until February 1983.[35]

Before moving on to a discussion of the scope of the pandemic in the region, I want to first put the arrival of AIDS in the region in direct conversation with the construction of the white heartland imaginary. The now thoroughly debunked narrative around the origins of HIV/AIDS, particularly in the United States in the early 1980s, was coalescing to somehow attribute to the virus a vaguely African origin that involved ingesting monkey blood, before it inexplicably spread to a gay Canadian flight attendant who then infected countless gay men on his flight routes between large coastal cities.[36] This narrative reinforced the white heartland imaginary in many ways: rural whiteness was as far from this origin as possible; immigrants and outlaws, particularly Black immigrants and gay men, were both villainized and expressly denied inclusion in the white heartland imaginary; and by making AIDS and the heartland seemingly incongruous, the region could remain the epitome of white strength, resilience, and vigor. However, Robert Rayford complicates all of this. The simple existence of Rayford's infection and death in 1969 shook national and global understandings of the epidemic's origins when news broke of the positive antibody test on nearly two-decades-old tissue in 1984.[37] However, the revelation's true potential to disrupt the early racist and homophobic narratives of the origins of AIDS never materialized as the slow onset of the pandemic in the region allowed for the reinforcement and perpetuation of the white heartland imaginary in the 1980s.

The number of cases of HIV/AIDS was dramatically smaller in the heartland, but not always to positive effect. To provide a clearer picture of the smaller case numbers, between 1982 and January 1989, only 531 cases of AIDS were reported in the entire Kansas City metropolitan area.[38] In 1985, Kansas City reported thirteen AIDS cases, while New York City reported nearly 3,000 cases.[39] While these numbers illustrate a true disparity of scope, they are also incomplete because they include cases of AIDS only, not HIV.[40] More problematically, these statistics do not capture the "coming home syndrome," a term that acknowledges that infections were counted at the site of diagnosis, not the patient's residence; thus, although some people moved post diagnosis from New York, for example, their cases were counted only in New York.[41] In this way, the erasure of AIDS from the heartland began with these initial methods of accounting for cases. The failure to acknowledge the "coming home syndrome" had significant implications for the heartland response, as state and federal funds (when they became available) were most commonly allocated based on an area's case numbers. In effect, this method of allocating funds consistently resulted in even less funding to address the needs of people with HIV/AIDS in the heartland region. Although those who were counted in the regional AIDS tally were not erased by reporting, their lives were made more precarious by the need to spread limited resources across a larger actual population whose needs had not been accounted for.

At the crux of the heartland response lies the issue of density—the density of medical infrastructure, and the density of the communities most impacted by HIV/AIDS. The heartland epidemic may have been smaller than the coastal epidemic in number of cases, but it was much larger in terms of geographic area, forcing local responses to cover areas spanning hundreds of miles for a handful of patients. The region also faced the epidemic with an anemic medical infrastructure. For example, cases in Kansas were spread out across a state that is about 400 miles long (roughly the distance from San Francisco to Los Angeles, or from Washington, DC, to Boston) and half as wide, with 105 counties, nearly 70 percent of which have between zero and twenty-five hospital beds in total. The western half of the state of Kansas, an area slightly smaller than the United Kingdom, had fewer than 200 hospital beds at the height of the AIDS crisis.[42] Simply getting to a doctor, let alone a doctor knowledgeable about HIV, could (and still can) often require a day or two and access to transportation. Added to these hurdles were the religiously and politically conservative communities that were both deeply insular and poorly educated about HIV/AIDS. Together, these obstacles to quality healthcare and home-making for people with HIV/AIDS appear as cliffs and mountains despite the notoriously flat landscape of the region.

Even though the number of cases in the heartland was relatively small, they were equally diverse in modes of transmission and populations impacted, and all spread out over a much larger area compared to cases in the coastal AIDS experience. The coal-mining southeastern portion of the region saw cases that originated from shared needles. Men having sex with men accounted for many cases in the towns as well as some scattered across the plains. Meatpacking towns and migrant farm laborers experienced HIV/AIDS spread via heterosexual sex in small and remote towns scattered across the heartland. Native American reservations (each with their complex histories and distrust of the US Indian Health Service) served as a backdrop to all modes of transmission.[43] Here, the reduced funds due to state and federal allocation formulas inflicted exponential pain, as efforts to provide for far-flung patients—which typically required long travel, additional outreach and education to multiple communities, and access to disparate care centers—all happened on very small budgets and with far fewer people (both paid and unpaid) to shoulder the labor. Any services of similar scope and scale to those provided by the Gay Men's Health Crisis of New York were only rarely or simply not possible in the heartland because there was not the density of gay men or of any other specific group disproportionately impacted by HIV/AIDS to warrant and run such an organization. Rather than building a web of new organizations and services born out of the AIDS crisis, activists and people with HIV/AIDS in the heartland instead had to piggyback on and transform as needed existing infrastructures of care in the region. In short, the heartland saw the confluence of multiple factors that led to community building or home-making that looked much different than it did on the coasts and cities.

Conclusion

Uncovering the history of AIDS in this region does the discursive work of naming the white heartland imaginary, but not to dismiss it or somehow make it evaporate like a toxic mist across the land. Rather, examining the early years of a horrible epidemic in the county's center makes visible the white heartland imaginary, a force that is invisible to many. By marking the white heartland imaginary and tracking it through a wide array of responses and a diverse cast of historical actors in the region, we gain a better understanding of not just the regional epidemic but also the social and political force of the white heartland imaginary that continues to shape our present and future. This history illuminates how the discursive construction of the white heartland imaginary serves as a tool, weapon, goal, and anathema, sometimes all at once. We gain greater clarity on how it is employed and deployed, and to what effect. Thus, the recounting of this overlooked history serves as both a lesson in history and a primer for this moment and going forward.

CHAPTER TWO

Trouble at Home

> There's no place like home.
> —DOROTHY, *The Wizard of Oz*

While the white heartland imaginary operates on a massive scale that coalesces in ways that impact individuals, the concept of home starts with the individual and works its way out to the larger community. The two concepts are intertwined and overlap, with the heartland white imaginary working as an overwhelmingly oppressive force for people with HIV/AIDS, and the contested concepts of home functioning as potential sites and forms of resistance. This chapter explores the concept of home within the white heartland imaginary in the early AIDS pandemic, particularly as it relates to an imagined sense of place, community, and belonging. To understand the history of HIV/AIDS in this region and its importance for the rest of the country, we must start with the paradoxical and contradictory position of home. At once, home can mean a specific place, a nostalgic feeling, a hope, an origin, a destination, a political mandate, a diasporic pitstop, an embodiment, and a constant reminder of freedoms denied or possible.

Among the roughly 50,000 panel blocks in the AIDS Memorial Quilt, there is one, #4227, that includes, among the eight panels in every block, a bright red panel with a simple, thin rainbow arching from one bottom corner to another, under which dark but fading lettering reads, "SOMEWHERE OVER THE RAINBOW LOVE LIVES ON." There is no name or geographic reference given on the panel itself. The reference to the famous song from *The Wizard of Oz* adds several possible layers to this particular quilt panel. Did the creators opt to include these words because the person they were memorializing was from Kansas, the backdrop of the movie, as a nod to a physical home? Or perhaps was the person a member of the gay community who idolized not only *The Wizard of Oz* but also Judy Garland, who played Dorothy and sang "Somewhere over the Rainbow" in an acknowledgment of a community that provided a sense of home? Perhaps the words commemorate a gay Kansan. Was the phrase not at all linked to *The Wizard of Oz* in the mind of the quilter; rather than referencing a ballad about home, perhaps the rainbow and wording speak to an afterlife or just a love of rainbows? Regardless, the quilter chose these words, colors, and imagery, specifically out of infinite other possibilities, to represent the person they memorialized in this fabric equivalent of a gravestone.

The context of the panel is what gives it meaning, but even this works in multiple ways. On the one hand, the context of the person memorialized and the quilter would reveal the meaning of the words and the rainbow in this individual panel, signifying a singular person as if to say, "This person was here." On the other hand, when placed as a single panel connected to a panel block of eight panels amid about 50,000 other panel blocks that together memorialize more than 100,000 people who have died of HIV/AIDS, the specific panel in panel block #4227 takes on an entirely different meaning. Here, the significance comes from the sheer number of deaths, as if to say, "This pandemic was here and killed so many." Adding more complexity and context to this single panel, many across the country, and particularly in the heartland, found the AIDS Quilt to be transformative in bringing education and humanity to the forefront of an epidemic that had bartered in ignorance and capitalized on dehumanizing those infected. In this context, it was as if the AIDS Quilt said, "You may not see people suffering, but human suffering cannot be denied in this." Meanwhile, many of the most vocal activists in various chapters of ACT UP criticized the AIDS Quilt for being too soft, too compromising, blunting both the rage and the critiques of the systems that propelled the epidemic, as if to say, "A quilt will not provide us healthcare or services."[1] Context matters in this singular quilt panel, in the AIDS Quilt as a whole, and in understandings of home.

Thinking about home in the heartland AIDS response is similar to tracing the different contexts of the panel in panel block #4227, in that historical actors do not declare themselves to be home among different groups of people or place a stake in the ground claiming a spot, just as the panel in block #4227 leaves a mystery about who is memorialized and why these specific words and a rainbow seemed most appropriate. Instead, home appears at times as discursive and at other times as material, but it is almost always contested. In this history, there is rarely agreement about who gets to be at home and what constitutes a home. For example, was a person who left the heartland for the coast, only to return once infected with HIV, coming home or leaving home? The answer might be different depending on whether you asked the returnee or members of the community to which they returned. What is the relationship to home for people who are shunned by the farming community that grounded their entire lives but find a new community of support through small-scale regional migration? In this instance, the concept of home varies by who defines it, whether the larger farming community, the new community, or the individual. Those actors who stayed, returned, or left the heartland are bound by two forces: the AIDS pandemic and the seismic, tectonic shift it brought to their understandings of home.

Again, like the specific panel in AIDS Quilt panel block #4227, home operates on the singular level (does a person with AIDS feel at home or have a space to call home) and on the systemic level. Home is the battleground for the white heartland imaginary. The ability to feel, create, and imagine a home is a critical piece in the operationalizing of the white heartland imaginary. The result of this combination of home and the heartland white imaginary creates Reagan's America in which neoliberalism, individuality, the rise of religion, conservatism, and the shrinking of the state's responsibilities become embedded with American identity. Only those who embody the white heartland imaginary feel truly at home in this iteration of America. These discourses are violent in that there are people who live in them who can never be or feel at home.

While the heartland region became the backdrop for the idealized white imaginary, its site as home for those most impacted by HIV/AIDS became increasingly complicated and contested during the arrival of the pandemic in the 1980s. The history of home in the heartland specifically reveals further complexity, especially when put against the backdrop of white settler colonialism. The arrival of AIDS in the heartland region combined with the erasing power of the white imaginary to render those most impacted homeless, at least discursively and temporarily, if not always materially and permanently.[2] After all, the physical region embodied the concept of the white heartland imaginary, and both the white heartland imaginary and the discourse of AIDS agreed—AIDS and those to blame for it are always somewhere other than the heartland. Amid the pandemic, those impacted by HIV/AIDS fell into one of three categories: those who stayed in the heartland to build communities locally, those who migrated to or within the heartland when previous homes became inhospitable or unsustainable, and those who fled the heartland to fight the pandemic in new communities. All three of these groups play central roles not only in shaping the history of HIV/AIDS in this region but also in informing the politics, coalitions, and tactics that would come to fuel much of the national LGBTQ, HIV-related, and racial politics of the late twentieth and early twenty-first centuries.

Each of these groups also experienced discursive homelessness and undertook the labor of home re-creation, revealing a complex definition of home that includes a sense of community that often defies a specific and singular space, identity, or region. In this way, the concept of "home" works similarly to the "floating signifier" that the philosophers Claude Lévi-Strauss, Jacques Derrida, and Jacques Lacan theorize to mean a signifier (such as a word, an image, or music) for which there is not a concrete referent. A floating signifier's meaning is garnered largely from its context, not unlike the specific panel in AIDS Quilt panel block# 4227. It can signify a singular person memorialized, a singular quilter, a song from a famous movie, gay culture, Kansas, the political power of the entire AIDS Quilt, its political softness in comparison to its contemporary ACT UP, and/or something else altogether. Stuart Hall uses the concept of a floating signifier to unpack race. He explains that "race works like a language . . . that is, it is always, or there is always, a certain sliding of meaning."[3] Evelynn Hammonds examined the floating signifiers of HIV/AIDS (though she didn't use that phrase) in her extensive work on HIV/AIDS in Black women in an era when it was assumed to be a white gay man's disease.[4] Douglas Crimp also took on the work of examining the various meanings attributed to the epidemic.[5] "Home" works similarly, particularly as it is simultaneously defined by several parties—the larger culture (here, the white heartland imaginary), members of the immediate surrounding community, those few deemed integral to home (often, one's family of origin), and the self. The context of the invocation and creation of home clarifies its meaning as a physical space, a community, feeling, aspiration, nostalgia, or something else entirely.

As the epidemic most impacted those already pushed outside the heartland ideals due to their race, sexuality, immigration status, or political posture, HIV/AIDS made claims to home in the region even more tenuous for them as the need for both a discursive and a material home increased dramatically in the shadow of sickness. The vast majority of those chronicled in this history lived outside of the imagined heartland ideal even as they lived in the geographic center of the country. The heartland AIDS history reveals home to be ephemeral, contested, unfixed, and deeply intertwined with other coexisting structures that are both imaginary and real—the nation, race, gender, sexuality, and class. Because the heartland is the imaginary white ideal of the 1980s that provides materiality to an imaginary communal white home, home in the heartland, particularly for those impacted by AIDS, illuminates the machinations of sexism, racism, homophobia, colonialism, class, and ableism inherent in an imagined home. In other words, the idea of the heartland was central to the very politics of retrenchment, family values, neoliberalism, and privatization that made life more tenuous for people impacted by HIV/AIDS who lived in the heartland.

The actual material making of home amid this inhospitable backdrop for those outside the white heartland imaginary but within its material borders provides insight into finding and crafting belonging when excluded. In other words, contesting and creating home when denied it proved to be central to HIV/AIDS organizing and resistance in the heartland. Through this lens, we gain clarity around the contours of racism, homophobia, and religious inflexibility. We also see a kind of queer home-making that spread far beyond queer communities to meet the needs of those written out of the heartland but still living within it. We see how discourses of the white heartland imaginary contributed to coastal and heartland communities while simultaneously eroding, erasing, or harming those who defied the construct. The power of the white heartland imaginary isolated the region from the larger AIDS narrative and denied a discursive home to those impacted, manifesting Reagan's America in the process. However, the tactics and politics deployed in the heartland AIDS response also shaped many political arenas beyond just HIV/AIDS: the LGBTQ political agenda of the late twentieth and early twenty-first centuries, the respectability politics at play within Black and immigrant communities, and the role of the Indian Health Service in denying the sovereignty of Native peoples.

Defining Home

Many of us understand home in the literal sense as the place to which we return at the end of the day, a place to rest, a site of refuge. It is here that we muddle the concept of homelessness when we mean unhoused. Home is both a physical space and an emotional, discursive one. Being homeless in one sense does not automatically translate to being homeless in the other. For example, to be unhoused means to lack a physical space but not necessarily to be without an emotional home. Meanwhile, being homeless discursively means the opposite—to be without (or to be denied) a sense of emotional belonging, regardless of access to material shelter. Offering a simplified but deeply emotional definition, Doris Davenport writes, "For me, home is a place where at least two things have happened: a minimal nurturing love and one positive experience that holds you in memory."[6] Home is also a central theme in much Latinx and Chicana feminist theory, particularly as they contemplate the border and borderlands and parse out the navigation and experience of multiple identities and cultures at once.[7] Gloria Anzaldúa argues in *This Bridge We Call Home: Radical Visions for Transformation* that "there are no safe spaces. 'Home' can be unsafe and dangerous because it bears the likelihood of intimacy and thus thinner boundaries. Staying 'home' and not venturing out from our group comes from woundedness and stagnates our growth. To bridge means loosening our borders, not closing off to others. Bridging is the work of opening the gate to the stranger, within and without."[8] This perspective adds greater complexity to understandings and definitions of home, placing great emphasis on seeking refuge and connection beyond home. As the AIDS pandemic descended, access to a discursive home often shifted; perhaps love was rescinded, or positive memories became tainted. Meanwhile, the need for sanctuary, a literal and material place to lie down, became a critical need for many infected with HIV/AIDS in the heartland. Attempts to meet this need while overcoming the new hurdles to home reveal a great deal about ideas of home, expectations of those who would need a home, and the underlying racial, economic, and sexual structures at work in the region.

Home, like the heartland and even HIV itself, straddles the imaginary and the real, the discursive and the material. These are all "floating signifiers."[9] While chapter 1 charted the imagined or discursive white heartland imaginary, I think it is also useful to unpack how HIV/AIDS similarly operates in the discursive and material realms. On the one hand, HIV and AIDS are supposedly easy to mark materially—whether one is infected or not, or immunocompromised to the extent of AIDS or not. We can see through a microscope whether HIV/AIDS exists materially or not. However, even within the clear epidemiological and infectious disease definitions, there is material wiggle room and debate. The definitions of HIV and AIDS have shifted over time to include a greater number of opportunistic infections (including gynecological ones), to reference the CD4 count, and to change the disease type from fatal to chronic. It now encompasses concepts like undetectability, new strains, and new prevention techniques. Add to that the widely uneven availability of medicines and preventatives, and the material experience of the disease is deeply tied to when, where, and who is infected.

The discourses around HIV/AIDS have had a significant impact on the definition, treatment, and lived experiences of those most impacted by the disease over the last forty years. These discourses are what nurture an entire burgeoning subfield of study that spans multiple disciplines. However, to provide an example of the discursive impact of the disease that goes far beyond a blood test or T-cell count, we need to look no further than the names and nicknames of the disease itself: initially, GRID (gay-related immune deficiency), then gay cancer, ARC (AIDS-related complex), the 4H disease (referring to hemophiliacs, homosexuals, Haitians, and heroin addicts, the four groups most closely tied to the early crisis), and finally HIV/AIDS. We could also explore the simple existence of AIDS phobia. AIDS phobia evokes images of harassment, public pool and bathroom closures, evictions, job insecurity, patients dying in hospital rooms where the doctors and nurses are afraid to touch them, and a lifetime of political, legal, and legislative battles. The discourse of AIDS combines with the materiality of AIDS to create the early AIDS crisis.

Similarly, home is both material and discursive: a feeling and a place, a site of nostalgia and longing for future manifestation, centered on individual embodiment while also tied to the communal. Home in the heartland, specifically during the early AIDS crisis, is both the imaginary home of possibility, stability, and belonging for much of the white population nationally (including those not physically situated in the heartland geography) and the material home of negotiated existence, communities of compromise, and subverting oppressive forces for those living in the region and touched by HIV/AIDS. The history of AIDS, more generally, is one in which, too often, the discursive claim to home and belonging vanishes or becomes fraught with infection. However, AIDS in the heartland specifically goes one step further, as many who were most impacted by the pandemic were already outside of the imagined white ideal in one way or another before the arrival of the virus. They were already experiencing home precarity on at least a discursive level. The pandemic made discursive barriers to home larger while simultaneously increasing the need for material and imagined home.

Centering this relationship to home and the white heartland imaginary serves two purposes. First, it uncovers an untold history of HIV/AIDS that is quite different from the existing historiography. But it goes further than simply filling a historiographical lacuna; it also propels theoretical understandings of home. The tactics developed to find home within a neoliberal political landscape combined with a material community in a thinly populated place reverberate outward from the heartland AIDS experience into the deployment of respectability politics among those groups disproportionately impacted by HIV/AIDS as well as the structural forms of racism, classism, ableism, and homophobia. AIDS in the heartland reveals home to be fleeting, imagined, and negotiated in a neoliberal nation-state marked by racism, classism, religiosity, ableism, homophobia, and conservatism. From this perspective, the history of AIDS in the heartland is equal parts examining the exclusion from home that many faced and the work of home-making under the duress of exclusion and infection.

This use of home and the definition of it as both material and discursive stands apart from a deeply personal or domestic kind of home. Stephen Vider, in his revelatory book *The Queerness of Home*, explores the importance of the deeply domestic spaces of the home and its role in gender, sexuality, and politics in the postwar period. With truly pathbreaking framing, he places home and domesticity at the center of his study, charting how movements and activism moved outward from the domestic spheres LGBTQ people created. For Vider, "Home has long been privileged in American life as a central site of intimate affiliation, a protected sphere where romance, marriage, and the family were imagined to find their deepest expression. . . . Lesbian, gay, bisexual, transgender, and queer people did not simply reproduce or reject such ideals but rather elaborated new domestic styles and intimacies as a primary means of negotiating their relationship to postwar sexual and gender norms and the nation."[10] My understanding of home is different. Home here is less about a physical domestic space and more about a sense of belonging, particularly in a region whose cultural construction excludes so many. This analysis also uses home to chart the history of a more diverse and expansive group of people whose identities overlapped with the LGBTQ identities but also expanded far beyond them. In this history, the heartland white imaginary, especially in concert with HIV/AIDS, denied a sense of home or a claim to belonging in the region for people in this group. But of course, they found and crafted new ways of belonging and new kinds of homes. In exploring this work of home-making, this book is in conversation with Vider's work.

Home in relationship to the act or feeling of belonging appears an important theoretical focal point in the heartland AIDS history. Belonging evokes a feeling of peace in the body, a supportive community, and easy access to care. AIDS in the heartland unsettles or interferes with belonging at every level. The realities of infection discipline the physical body in terms of viral loads and symptoms, but also in terms of how people with AIDS discipline or police themselves to gain proximity to belonging.[11] When a gay son returns from San Francisco to the family farm infected, familial and community support often relied on secrecy or "toning it down" in a way that swaps one kind of unbelonging for another form of unbelonging. Dr. Donna Sweet recounted this chilling story of one of her first patients with HIV: "One of the first Sundays he was home, he went to church with his folks. And that afternoon, the minister called and said, 'You are welcome to come back, but he is never to darken our door again, we are fumigating the church as we speak.'"[12] The history of AIDS in the heartland is a history of looking for or making home, seeking belonging, and building an approximation in its absence.

Rendered Homeless at Home

Jay Johnson first encountered HIV/AIDS toward the end of his undergraduate career at the University of Kansas, which he attended from 1983 to 1986. As a member of the campus group Gay and Lesbian Students of Kansas (GLSOK), the equivalent of the student gay-straight alliance, he found himself involved in HIV/AIDS educational programs and events. Amid the safe-sex education programs and educational panels with local public health officials, Johnson learned in 1986 that a close family friend who had recently returned home from living in New York had passed away from the disease. There were many similar stories of becoming infected in big cities and returning to the heartland associated with a significant portion of AIDS deaths in the region at the time, and they would become quite familiar to Johnson in the coming years. A gay Kansan of Native American descent, he had never really left his physical home region. Yet, his life after graduation certainly demonstrates the way that the landscape of home shifted under his feet.

After graduation, Johnson secured a job as a bank teller, which he quickly realized was not what he wanted to do: "I worked 366 days before I left." Against the backdrop of the AIDS crisis, which had been recently illustrated by the spreading of the AIDS Quilt across the National Mall in Washington, DC, in October 1987, and with the activism of his undergraduate years fresh in his mind, he opted to pursue a master's degree in social welfare at the University of Kansas in order to help AIDS patients and people with HIV in the region.[13] Though people at the university and in his personal life advised against getting too involved with AIDS, Johnson began volunteering in 1989 at what would shortly become the Topeka AIDS Project. The volunteering quickly filled in every available gap in his schedule as he also juggled full-time coursework, the related practicum at the Topeka Veterans Affairs hospital, and, at times, other jobs to help pay the rent. Topeka, about thirty minutes to the west of Lawrence, soon became the more logistically feasible place to live, though Lawrence remained where he felt at home. As a result, he left his physical hometown of Lawrence and moved west to Topeka. Those thirty minutes, which covers as many miles, matter in the Kansas landscape, especially for a gay Native man—Topeka is the capital city of deeply conservative Kansas, a bigger city and much grittier than Lawrence, which is the blue bastion of the state, anchored by the University of Kansas and Haskell

Indian Nations University, complete with a downtown strip dotted with restaurants and boutiques that wouldn't thrive anywhere else in the state. The short drive across mostly flat terrain traversed a political chasm.

While working with and for people with HIV/AIDS, he witnessed repeated moments of ejection, rejection, and denial of home for those who were HIV-positive. He saw this from multiple angles as he scrambled to meet the vast needs of the Topeka AIDS project. He recalled in an interview, "Topeka AIDS Project was a single office in the Topeka Shawnee County Health Department. They were giving us office space because we were picking up the slack when they were getting positive test results."[14] The organization, though responsible for providing services to people all over northeast Kansas, from Manhattan and Junction City up to Nebraska, relied solely on volunteers, mostly "middle-aged and elderly lesbians who were part of MCC," until Johnson was offered a part-time paid position in late 1989. For reference, in terms of the national experience of HIV/AIDS, by this point, ACT UP was in its heyday, national infections hovered around 115,000 cases, and the major medicine prescribed to treat HIV remained AZT, which proved highly toxic for many. The initial caseload at the Topeka AIDS Project, all Johnson's responsibility, hovered around twenty-five patients before jumping to well over 100 in the next few years. Johnson began as a community volunteer counselor, meaning that "we were either in the room when they got the results, or we were brought in right afterward. . . . People weren't getting tested until they were sick. . . . About half were people who had moved home, and about half were people who were in Kansas and were diagnosed in Kansas." Often, it was in these counseling sessions immediately after diagnosis that Johnson first witnessed a loss of home for those with HIV/AIDS. In those conversations, he helped navigate people through the feeling of betrayal by their physical bodies, followed shortly by imagining the immediate and midterm future in which access to physical home was often made or assumed to be more precarious by their diagnosis.

While complex and emotional, these conversations were just the start of Johnson's work, as he became the catalyst for connecting hardly existent services to patients who were growing in number and need. Beyond offering a Kleenex box and sitting with folks through their diagnosis, Johnson's work included driving from one client to another across hundreds of miles, educating locals about HIV, and negotiating care for those who needed it. Then, he began manifesting new relationships to home for those rendered homeless, either physically or discursively, due to their HIV status. After earning his master's degree in social welfare in 1991, Johnson became the organization's first executive director and hired two additional employees. Together, they offered individual counseling, support groups, and hospital visitations to help foster a sense of peace, belonging, and acceptance—in short, they sought to build a sense of home for HIV-positive people within their bodies and in new and existing communities.

Crafting a pathway to a discursive home was only part of the work of reimagining home. Johnson hustled behind the scenes to ensure material homes and wrangle for care, cajoling hospital beds, battling to get medications covered by Medicaid, and writing grants to pay for the services as well as his salary. The work was all-consuming and relentless. Illuminating the desperation of the local situation, he explained, "There were no hospice or nursing home placements. No nursing home or hospice anywhere in the region would accept AIDS patients."[15] However, a brief memory of a "funny" conversation with a Topeka doctor, one of only three who had agreed to even see HIV-positive patients in northeast Kansas, shone a spotlight on how big of role he and the other Topeka AIDS Project workers played in getting services for those who needed them: "I was begging him, begging him to take on a client. 'You know my track record! They will have Medicaid. You will not be left hanging for payment! I will kiss your feet!' And he was like, 'Please don't.'"[16] Here, Johnson explains how a patient's access to medical care hinged on his relationships with individual providers.

Through the lens of home, Johnson's career became about little else, even as it had so many facets. Large portions of his day were often dedicated to finding a physical space or beds for people, while much of the rest of the day was spent creating a sense of community and belonging among HIV-positive people or educating the larger community in the hope that it would become less unhospitable to his clients. He did all of this while removed—if only by a thirty-minute drive—from the town he felt was his own home. Furthermore, the pressure of the constant, high-stakes negotiations with providers, patients, and different communities made Johnson's health falter, and his most basic, embodied sense of home started to strain.

By the fall of 1993, Johnson had found his way home to Lawrence, alleviating some of his personal feelings of disrupted home, but the physical and emotional strain in his body continued as he shifted jobs within the AIDS service sector. As part of his work with the Topeka AIDS project, he regularly did educational and prevention events with local Indian nations, particularly the Kickapoo, and collaborated with Haskell Indian Nations University. A person in management from the National Native American AIDS Prevention Center (NNAPC, pronounced "napsy") attended one such training and on the spot, offered Johnson a job to become the director of client services for the national organization. Founded in 1987, NNAPC was the only HIV-specific Native American organization in the country, and the first Native American health organization funded entirely outside of the Indian Health Service and Bureau of Indian Affairs. This new position allowed him to fully focus his attention on the AIDS epidemic among Native nations, of which he himself was a member (Delaware and Cherokee). Though he regularly had to travel to Oklahoma, Arizona, and the Western mountain states, ironically, the job at NNAPC allowed him to move back to his home of Lawrence, Kansas, for the first time in several years.

HIV/AIDS among Native people offers a window into additional layers of contested notions of home. The concept of home for Native nations and communities is deeply fraught even without the addition of HIV/AIDS, as continued US colonization and the historically violent annexation of land have removed many Native communities from their original homelands, forcibly relocated them to reservations that are often characterized by poorly resourced lands, and overly policed and abused them both off and on reservation lands. Because many Native cultures place great religious and cultural significance on the relationship with the earth and land, these territorial violations take on a compounded discursive and material meaning of homelessness. To this already burdened battle for home, issues of health and sickness added many more layers. Most healthcare among Native communities, beyond traditional Native medical practices, relies on the Indian Health Service, a federally funded program that offers free and low-cost health services to members of recognized Native nations for many basic healthcare needs. However, the Indian Health Service inherited significant historical baggage from centuries of mistreatment of Native peoples by white colonizers, starting with the British distributing blankets infested with smallpox in 1763 and continuing to the present, where there are still cases of forced sterilizations and ongoing trauma in Indian Health Service facilities. Many Native communities view the Indian Health Service with a great deal of skepticism and suspicion but often do not have easy access to other healthcare. In terms of home, there were many patients in Indian Health Service examination rooms who were already forcibly displaced from ancestral material homes and worried for their bodily autonomy and sovereignty. HIV/AIDS compounded these problems and added to them the stigma of the disease, the misinformation, and the miscounting of cases. Johnson remembered, "There'd been a few studies early on that showed that the HIV rate among Native Americans was a hidden epidemic because a lot of people were being reported as Hispanic or white and not as Native American, so there was a big push to rectify that."[17] Additionally, early on, AIDS was seen as a white gay man's disease. Combined with the significant stigma people with HIV/AIDS faced, the need for education and intervention among these communities was great.[18]

Johnson's professional life became focused on giving aid to those rendered not just homeless but nonexistent by the heartland white imaginary, along with other structurally violent formations. The Ahalya Project in Oklahoma, one of the many projects he worked on, was dedicated to making visible the true state of the AIDS epidemic among Native communities. He organized testing drives, support groups, and prevention programs for Native communities across the region. With significant funding from the federal Health Resources and Services Administration, Johnson's days were less about haggling for care, temporary housing, and building homes for those rejected from or denied their previous homes. Instead, he grappled with home on a larger structural scale in which Native people are constantly denied their homes, are rendered invisible, and face complex decisions and numerous barriers to staying on or leaving the reservation. To navigate this complex landscape of home, Johnson and NNAPC embraced the power of Native people working for and with other Native people in response to HIV/AIDS. Working around and beyond the Indian Health Service's complicated and painful history with respect to most Native peoples, the concept of peer education and care resonated significantly, expanding the contested notions of home at work in Native communities to include knowledge and conversations about HIV/AIDS. Johnson taught a peer education course in 1994 at Haskell University that included prevention, education, and care.

His relationship with Haskell remained intact even as Johnson transitioned in 1994 into a position as the state HIV/AIDS coordinator for the Kansas Department of Health. By this point, AZT had gained approval for use in fetal HIV as the national HIV/AIDS narrative saw a significant uptick in pediatric AIDS cases.[19] Over 270,000 people had died from AIDS in the United States, and the Ryan White CARE Act of 1990 was infusing more government funding into all aspects of AIDS research. With his new position, Johnson's frame of home changed again to encompass the entire state as his work blended the skills he had acquired at the Topeka AIDS Project and as the NNAPC director of client services. However, the political landscape was also shifting by that time, as Democratic governor Joan Finney lost to the much more conservative Republican Bill Graves later that year. With Graves would come a full about-face on the state's involvement and support of sex education, AIDS prevention and services, and even access to abortion. I will explore this political shift more in the next chapters, but here it suffices to say that the ethos of the Summer of Mercy, a series of anti-abortion protests in Wichita in the summer of 1991, had spread into every corner of the social and political fabric of Kansas by late 1994. The result was that people impacted by HIV/AIDS were often rendered both materially and discursively homeless with greater frequency, violence, and political support than before, and the act of home-making became harder.

As the new governor took office in 1995, Johnson stepped back from his career in AIDS work. Exhausted and burnt out, having spent so much energy and time fighting for an approximation of home for others, he had alienated himself from his own body. He took the discovery of the HAART treatment in 1996 as his permission to leave home and the work of home-making to remake himself. He moved to Seattle and then attended graduate school in Hawaii to study geography, eventually returning to Kansas to be a professor of geography and atmospheric sciences as well as Indigenous studies at the University of Kansas. Though previously he had continuously lived within a fifty-mile radius, his relationship with home had transformed over the decade of his involvement with AIDS services, so much so that to reclaim some sense of self and home, he had had to move far away and completely change career trajectories before he could reimagine a home for himself back in the heartland.

Johnson is one of many who stayed in the heartland in the face of AIDS but simultaneously was rendered discursively homeless. He had found hard-fought success in providing many others with shelter and communities in which they could claim some proximity to home, but this work, its difficulty, and the discrimination it laid bare made him feel more alienated from the heartland. This alienation and physical and emotional exhaustion provide insight into the inner workings of the white heartland imaginary and the importance of contesting home. By making home precarious, uncomfortable, and constantly contested, the white heartland imaginary flexed its power, not just by making those who did not meet the ideals of the white heartland imaginary want to leave, but also by making any attempt to circumvent the neoliberalism it venerated exhausting, demoralizing, and ultimately a failure of individuals rather than the state. Jay Johnson gives a clear window into these maneuverings, which were happening on a national scale as society became more convinced by the neoliberal tropes of pulling yourself up by the bootstraps and caring for yourself and ostracizing or villainizing anyone who couldn't or wouldn't.

Home Refugees

In 1988, Michael Edland, a well-regarded interior designer in St. Louis, cajoled many of his designer friends and wealthy clients to donate antiques and valuable furniture pieces to sell in a garage sale, a three-day, high-end fundraiser for which Edland designed a showroom in the parking garage of St. Louis's luxurious Plaza Frontenac, a mall anchored by Saks Fifth Avenue. The event raised $40,000 for DOORWAYS, a nonprofit tasked with providing housing for people with AIDS in St. Louis, Missouri. The funds, along with significant financial contributions from Catholic Charities, the Jewish Foundation, and the major service and funding arms of a handful of Protestant denominations, went to refurbishing a donated dilapidated building on the city's racial dividing line, Delmar Boulevard, on St. Louis's Northside.[20]

In rehabilitating the building, envisioned as a mixture of a "country club and fraternity house" for gay men dying of AIDS with nowhere else to go, Edland's volunteer designer team used a donated piano, bookshelves, and thick cushioned armchairs to create warm and comfortable communal spaces for imagined young men suddenly faced with the physical capacities of much older and infirm men.[21] According to many recollections, just as they "finished fluffing the last decorative pillow and opened the space" for the AIDS "fraternity house," a low-income Black woman and her two children walked in as their first residents.[22] They had just arrived in St. Louis, having been forced to migrate with one-way bus tickets bought with pooled funds from their fearful neighbors in a small rural town in southeast Missouri; each of them had just one suitcase. "That was it, that was all they had," recalled one DOORWAYS founding board member.[23] The new resident, Pat (not her real name), recalled in a 1988 interview, "I can't tell you what my life would be like without DOORWAYS because I can't even bring myself to think about it."[24]

Pat and her children turned the vision Edland had had for potential residents on its head, illuminating how even homes (both material and discursive) created specifically for those rendered homeless by the AIDS epidemic could, and often did, still echo exclusionary aspects of the white heartland imaginary. Pat's arrival signifies the infections among Black women (and people of color generally) that hit *simultaneously* with the emergence of AIDS among gay men in the region, challenging the often whitewashed origins of AIDS that focus entirely on white gay communities and defying the white heartland imaginary.[25]

Pat's experience demonstrates the recurring loss and reimagining of home that occurred in the heartland for those touched by the AIDS crisis. Pat's arrival at DOORWAYS exemplifies partial belongings, having been driven from one home that denied her because of her infection to a new home that was built for entirely different residents. The one-way bus ticket out of her hometown was a purchase born of fear, not compassion, a communal excision rather than an act of mutual aid for a neighbor with HIV.[26] Pat's story is far from unique. AIDS precipitated all different kinds of migration by those impacted by the pandemic, one form of which was forced. Regional migration from rural areas into urban centers both for care and at the insistence of AIDS-phobic communities became a hallmark of the heartland AIDS experience, as one interview revealed, "They either moved here for services or were brought here and dumped."[27] Physically moving from one home and arriving at another that was built for someone else makes for a complicated relationship to a discursive home and sense of belonging. Pat's story illuminates how gender, race, poverty, and parenthood combined with HIV status to repeatedly deny easy access to home in both the discursive and material senses.

Pat's response also reveals the roles of respectability, neoliberalism, and heteronormativity in navigating such an inhospitable landscape and negotiating some form of home for her and her family. As one of the first residents, Pat became a voice and face of the organization, frequently attending fundraisers and featuring prominently in promotional materials and fundraising videos. While she may not have been what Edland had imagined, the space he created did come to offer a sense of home to Pat and her children, or so she regularly professed at DOORWAYS events. Pat passed away long before I began this research, and her children have scattered. As a result, I want to be careful not to put words in her mouth. However, I do think it is worthwhile to put her work into a larger context of a regional sense of individualism, a national narrative of neoliberalism in which self-sufficiency is critical to avoid failure, and firmly in the shadow of the white heartland imaginary.[28] Her involvement in fundraising for DOORWAYS reflects not only a sense of discursive home she potentially fostered through living in one of the organization's buildings but also an exchange of labor for services, a sort of earning a physical home she could otherwise be denied. We have no way of knowing if this was part of her calculus in her vocal support for the organization, but we can note that both the organization and Pat were deeply enmeshed in a neoliberal system that expects a form of payment for everything and a white imaginary that placed the poor, Black, HIV-positive single mother firmly outside the norm. In chapter 3 we will examine how the assumed straightness of Pat became central in a larger respectability narrative on which DOORWAYS and much of the regional AIDS response relied.

AIDS migrations in the region extended beyond the rural surroundings as gay men returned to the Midwest in their final months of life and often in dire financial and medical situations, as their coastal gay enclaves could no longer support them. Migration played an important role in the heartland epidemic and response. A growing literature has documented the role of urban centers in the definition of LGBTQ communities and cultures, both currently and in the past. Whether observed by John D'Emilio in "Capitalism and Gay Identity" in the early 1980s or theorized by Scott Herring more recently, cities have long offered greater financial independence, anonymity, and the promise of a sexual community, drawing many from small towns and rural places to bigger, coastal cities.[29] Indeed, nearly half of those I interviewed for this book spoke of relocating to larger cities either within the heartland or on the coasts. However, as the pandemic took hold in cities like New York and Los Angeles, many who had migrated to the coasts and created new homes and communities faced new factors that pushed them back to the heartland. As an AIDS activist who moved to St. Louis from Washington, DC, in 1987 explained, "In DC, we were losing, I mean we were attending one funeral a month, no, a week, even! It was really hard for us . . . because we were losing so many friends."[30] Some returned to the heartland preemptively out of fear for their health as word of the pandemic spread, while others journeyed back only when their coastal social communities had collapsed, when few other options remained, or, often, as their health declined.[31] The first case of HIV/AIDS seen in the state of Kansas fell into this latter category, in the form of a young man who was brought to the hospital by his family on their way home from picking him up at the airport.[32] The vast majority of these people had not planned to return to the heartland when they did, and some of them, not at all.[33] They had left the region for a variety of reasons—in search of fun, school, work, community, or relief from family and small communities or religious and political conservatism. The pandemic changed their calculus. As the only physician in the region with a specialty in HIV and AIDS, Donna Sweet of Wichita explained: "Oftentimes, people who had grown up around here went to the coasts to experience a freer lifestyle, acquired [HIV]/AIDS, and ended up destitute and needing help, so they would come back to the homeland for help."[34]

Returning home sometimes meant moving back in with families of origin. The family receptions were as varied as the individual relationships we all have with family: some were welcomed back with open arms, some were welcomed only if they kept their identities and illnesses hidden from local community members, and others were forced back into the closet as they hid their identities in exchange for palliative care. A small number left their doctors to reveal their diagnoses to family members after hospitalization or even death, as mentioned above.[35] Interestingly, some returned to their home regions with no intention of engaging with their families of origin.[36] In these instances, people chose to migrate to the heartland out of desperation, heartbreak, and burnout from the devastation they experienced on the coasts. Chuck Gulas explained his hesitation in getting involved in AIDS activism after relocating to St. Louis: "The burnout when you are working in a crisis organization like that is very, it's very hard."[37] Whether in terms of their depleted T-cells or suffering in the throes of grief and rage, those who returned to the heartland had been severely harmed by HIV/AIDS and came to the heartland for solace and reprieve and a new home, despite the heartland white imaginary posting a "not welcome" sign.

Here again, the machinations of the white heartland imaginary become clear. The white heartland imaginary created a shared imagined, valorized ideal and villainized any other reality. Against this backdrop, the sense of belonging and home became the fulcrum on which this idea was leveraged, creating a strong sense of belonging for those in line with the ideal and significant discomfort (both emotional and physical) for those who challenged it. Both a sense of belonging in this carefully constructed concept of home and the fear of expulsion from it led many to embrace a series of governmental policies that became the backbone of neoliberalism and Christian conservative thought, even though these policies were harmful to the majority of people.

In Search of Home

A smaller number of interviewees for this project moved away from the heartland to coastal cities in response to the unsettling of home in the heartland, which provides another opportunity to explore how the heartland white imaginary combined with the arrival of HIV in the region to alter understandings of home.[38] Push and pull factors significantly shaped the decision to leave the heartland. As word of the intensity of the early epidemic on the coasts spread to the heartland, a handful of people found that home for them was tied more to identity than to location. These few stand out as anomalies among what Clare Forstie calls the "ambivalent communities" of LGBTQ folks in the Midwest.[39] If we accept Forstie's argument that LGBTQ identity-based community building and activism is blunted by large-scale ambivalence in the region, those who left the heartland for the coasts amid the early pandemic are rare exceptions, equivalent to the firefighter who runs into the burning building as everyone else flees.

Bill LaRock and Cathy Johnson met in 1987 when they both responded to an advertisement in the *St. Louis Post-Dispatch* for volunteers for the recently founded St. Louis Effort for AIDS (EFA), which LaRock succinctly explained was "kind of the St. Louis version of the Gay Men's Health Crisis" in New York. Drawing on his training as a psychiatric nurse, he developed a case management system for EFA and also led a grief group for survivors.[40] Meanwhile, Cathy used her skills as a social worker to step in as the volunteer director of social services for the organization. The two became fast friends, along with Bill's partner Glen. Cathy was inspired to do more in the fight against AIDS, having recently returned from Washington, DC, where she attended the March on Washington and saw the AIDS Quilt laid out on the Mall. She remembered, "It had a huge impact. . . . The NAMES Project was very political then." In addition to his work with EFA, Johnson also became deeply involved in the NAMES Project, as did Bill. When the quilt made its first national tour in 1988, it arrived in St. Louis in April of that year, and LaRock and Johnson befriended the NAMES Project volunteers who were traveling from San Francisco to escort the quilt. For nearly three years, the two juggled their activism in EFA and the NAMES Project along with full-time jobs and relationships, not to mention the increasing care required by sick friends. However, there was a growing undertone of frustration for both of them. LaRock recalled, "There was so much stigma, you know, stigma, fear. I had friends who waited years before they got tested because they were afraid of the results, they were afraid of who would find out, they were afraid of losing their jobs, they were afraid of their health insurance companies finding out. . . . The continued lack of resources and government support hadn't improved much from day one. Our growing frustration for the lack of attention and resources led us on this journey to start something that was more direct and more expressive of our continued outrage."[41] In the late 1980s, ACT UP seemed to be the most useful outlet for AIDS outrage, as chapters on the coast became known for their creative and disruptive forms of protest against a wide array of institutions, from the government and government agencies to the Catholic Church, and from pharmaceutical companies to Wall Street.

Starting in August 1990, LaRock and Johnson took out an advertisement in the local gay newspaper: "ACT UP St. Louis is coming." Johnson recalled, "It came out of a place of frustration and anger, feeling just paralyzed and watching people die."[42] On Monday, August 27, 1990, Bill and Cathy sat on stools in the Sunshine Inn, a vegetarian restaurant in St. Louis's Central West

End, as they waited to meet the founding members of ACT UP St. Louis. Not many people showed up. Johnson remembered ten to fifteen, while LaRock recalls a number closer to five—"We had a hard time attracting people."[43] Regardless, they talked about nonviolent direct action and came up with some ideas for future protests, planning their first for September 11 at the Social Security Administration to demand that AIDS-related and defining infections qualify for presumptive disability for Social Security. They held several actions in the following months at City Hall, the Department of Health, and the Social Security Administration building, to name a few of the sites. As a result, "we felt empowered in some ways and did some useful stuff but always with 'gosh, will there ever be more than twelve of us?'"[44]

These protests and actions were all part of a much larger ACT UP Change the Definition campaign across the country that aimed to expand the CDC definition of AIDS to include a greater number of opportunistic infections (including gynecological) and a CD4 count that, in turn, would entitle many more people to disability benefits and protections from housing and employment discrimination on account of their infection. The national campaign took more than two years and included a class action lawsuit, *S. P. v. Sullivan*, before finally manifesting change. Locally, protests at least felt more impactful for Cathy, as she explained, "In a certain way, we affected some changes in St. Louis that couldn't happen in the larger cities. In St. Louis, a die-in, laying on the street . . . that was big news. That was no longer a big deal in New York unless you blocked Fifth Avenue or St. Patrick's Cathedral." She was right; protests made headlines for several days in the local press, and "we didn't even go inside!"[45] St. Louis ACT UP was successful at raising the issue, heightening awareness, and often making local officials and government workers bend to their demands in whatever ways they could on the very local scale.

Despite the success of the small group of activists, LaRock and Johnson were taken aback by the response they received from other AIDS organizations. LaRock spoke with clarity when he recalled, "It did not sit well with nice gay and lesbian folks who had built this nice community-based organization [EFA]. . . . I think we were both a little surprised by the fear and animosity it created." Both knew that the tactics of ACT UP were a more radical approach to AIDS activism, but neither anticipated it eliciting such a response. LaRock explained, "EFA wouldn't let us meet in their office space. It became sort of a big deal. Half of the board resigned. They had allowed us to meet in their space a couple of times, and then they kicked us out. We hadn't even done anything public yet, but they were worried about offending people, sensibilities, all that stuff, all that Midwestern stuff." Within a year of its founding, St. Louis ACT UP had folded and both LaRock and Johnson had moved to San Francisco in hopes of being with their friends from the NAMES Project. Sadly, "most of them actually died before we got there," but LaRock and Johnson stayed because they "just wanted to live somewhere where gay people were not second-class citizens."[46] The same fate befell the tiny ACT UP chapters in Topeka, Kansas City, and Omaha: They were anemic in numbers and not welcomed by the larger local AIDS movement, and they often closed with their leaders leaving town for the coasts.

Here we see the power of the white heartland imaginary at work in the way that it policed the actions and expectations of not just the larger communities but also the gays and lesbians and others on the front lines of the regional AIDS response. LaRock traced the power of the heartland white imaginary, though he called it "Midwestern sensibilities":

> The idea that it [ACT UP] would be in the Midwest offended a lot of people's sensibilities of how to do things. In general, but even within the gay and lesbian community. When EFA hired their first CEO, or whatever the title was, they hired a straight, religious woman because they were afraid of hiring a gay man. It was the whole, "Yes, we know we're gay, but let's not shout it, let's work on the sympathy angle. We don't want to upset the straight people." They were trying to attract state and local foundation grants, that kind of thing. So they were trying to kind of keep the HIV world and the gay world separate. . . . They didn't want to offend people. They could generate sympathy for sick people but not for gay people.

As a result, LaRock and Johnson felt the pull to help address the bigger crisis on the coasts but also, more importantly, to be among like-minded activists. However, the push factor of being villainized by the organization they had been so influential in from the start and pegged as destructive forces in the local AIDS response proved integral in their decisions to move. Somewhat ironically, both LaRock and Johnson moved to San Francisco hoping to step back from AIDS-specific work and into larger lesbian and gay community building. Shortly after their arrival, they both became deeply entwined in gay and lesbian AIDS activism. LaRock said, "I didn't plan on making HIV my life's work, but it has been since then."[47]

In placing LaRock and Johnson's experience into the larger conversation about home and belonging amid the AIDS crisis in the heartland white imaginary, two major points emerge. First, the AIDS Quilt deserves more attention here. Scholar Marika Sturken wrote on the paradox of the quilt on the Mall,

"The quilt form evokes a sense of Americana, yet it also represents those who have been symbolically excluded from America—drug users, blacks, Latinos, gay men."[48] The quilt embraces a texture and art form tightly associated with the heartland to acknowledge those the heartland erases. It embodies the battle for material and discursive home that played out for those touched by HIV/AIDS in the heartland. Seeing the quilt on display, both in full on the National Mall and in the segments that traveled across the country, was a touchstone that spurred personal activism for many people interviewed for this book, not just Cathy and Bill. While many members of ACT UP chapters on the coasts derided the quilt as softening critiques of the state and evoking the tragedy rather than the rage of the epidemic, those far removed from coastal fury often found the quilt a consciousness-raising, activism-igniting, and perspective-transforming tool that worked with great efficacy in the heartland. From the perspective of the heartland, the AIDS Quilt takes on a much more catalyzing role than the more passive display and consumption of grief often depicted in the larger national history of AIDS.

Second, LaRock and Johnson's story charts another form of home denied or made inhospitable in the wake of AIDS in the heartland. Here, the loss of their discursive homes and communities was not due to illness, forced relocation, or even family rejection. While Bill and Cathy saw the quagmire of AIDS as a reason to embrace more radical and emotional forms of protest, it seems that the larger AIDS movement in the region came to a completely different conclusion, and it tightened its tactical grip on respectability, assimilation, and politeness. This disconnect ultimately ruptured the discursive and material relationship to home both for LaRock and Johnson and for ACT UP. These political migrants followed in the path of other regional trailblazers who had started in the heartland before moving to the coasts to find a broader audience and political spectrum. Though they are rarely claimed by heartland history, two founders of the Sisters of Perpetual Indulgence (a San Francisco–based charity, street performance, and protest organization) hailed from Iowa, Cleve Jones (co-founder of the NAMES Project AIDS Memorial Quilt) was from Indiana, and Phyllis Lyon (co-founder of the Daughters of Bilitis) started in Tulsa, Oklahoma.[49] For these activists, the politics of the moment (early homophile activism, gay liberation, or the AIDS crisis) recalibrated their relationships with home. Home became less about geography or origin and more about sexuality and the desire to create and care for an identity-based community. Here again, the white heartland imaginary tactfully deployed its ideas of home to push those who do not fit in or do not subscribe to the white heartland imaginary into the few geographic locations in the country that fell beyond the banner of the heartland, solidifying the notion that all of the United States endorsed the white heartland imaginary and the neoliberalism and political conservatism it signified. Even as I make this point, I want to be very clear that political radicalism existed in the heartland throughout the AIDS epidemic and still exists today. However, it thrives in different spaces and under different banners than those often found on the coasts, a topic explored more in chapter 5.

Conclusion

These first two chapters have charted the destructive power of the white heartland imaginary and the AIDS pandemic against those most impacted by the disease. The following chapters will shift to examine what forms of home, activism, medicine, and politics thrived in this region in the shadow of the white heartland imaginary. The HIV/AIDS epidemic reorganized communities by pulling some back to a community they had left for other regions, forcing new kinds of collaborations and interreliance among some existing but historically insular communities, and pushing others out of the heartland altogether to find new communities. All of this contestation of home was an integral piece in the creation and maintenance of the white heartland imaginary and the larger conservative and neoliberal swing of the 1980s and 1990s.

The work of building a heartland AIDS response amid the shifts in home and the shadow of the white heartland imaginary echoes many concepts introduced by queer futurity, the assembling of assemblages, the limitations of embodiment, and the machinations of race, diaspora, migration, and citizenship on the body.[50] The following chapters explore the ways that material resource distribution reflects discourses on who is valuable, who belongs, and who is deserving, which are tightly interwoven with race, gender, sex, disease, and politics, and how that distribution of resources is subverted and rerouted by activists who themselves fall outside the boundaries of those deemed valuable, belonging, or worthy. Examining the creation of an AIDS response in the heartland charts the creation of discursive and material homes for and by those initially rendered homeless by the arrival of the epidemic in the heartland and by the white heartland imaginary. This contestation of home played a central role in the larger political shifts of the 1980s and 1990s as it paved the way for the white heartland imaginary to take hold, for conservatism and neoliberalism to suffuse the national culture and shift the entire political spectrum of the nation rightward. Focusing on home highlights the mechanics of this shift and the efforts to thwart it.

CHAPTER THREE

Religion
The Politics of Piety

Much like the various praying hands monuments that dot the region, including the one pictured below by Earl Iversen (figure 3.1), religion looms large over nearly every aspect of the heartland, including the AIDS response. The social and political landscape of the entire heartland region is steeped in religion, which also colored, and even instigated, much of the AIDS response. It binds the fabric of the heartland white imaginary, constructions, and contestations of home and conjures the material regional AIDS response. Religion itself lives at the intersection of the material and imagined; religion allows people to affiliate with one another to build material buildings, communities, and services for one another based on a shared belief and faith in an intangible God. In the heartland, the relationship between religious institutions and a coordinated regional AIDS response was nothing short of integral. One person who served on numerous St. Louis AIDS-related boards stated that without religious organizations, "there would not have been any response" to AIDS in St. Louis.[1] Though nonreligious responses did exist, they were certainly meager by comparison and regularly interwoven into religious outreach or services.

Religion played a vastly different role in the heartland AIDS response than it is depicted to have played in much of the coastal-focused AIDS historiography. In AIDS histories focused on the coasts, or most AIDS historiography, religion rarely appears except as having been obstructionist at best and a tool for mass-produced bigotry and homophobia at worst. Perhaps the most obvious example of this is the 1989 Stop the Church campaign, in which ACT UP New York activists staged several protests against the Catholic Church's response to the AIDS epidemic (specifically, its stance against condoms and safe sex), most famously disrupting a mass held by Cardinal John O'Connor with a die-in and then vocal protests. That particular action resulted in over forty arrests.[2] Of course, religious organizations along the coasts played important positive roles in the pandemic response as well, but those stories often get left out or relegated to brief nods to individual institutions or organizations in the larger historiography, except in a handful of books that explore religion specifically.[3] The major exception to this is the Shanti

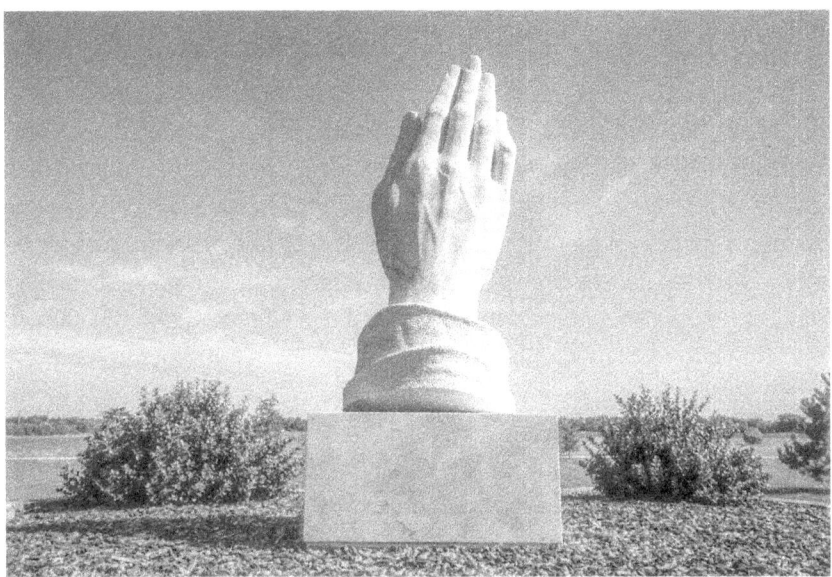

FIGURE 3.1 Earl Iversen, *Praying Hands Monument, Graveyard, Route 54, Wichita, 1976*. Vintage gelatin silver print. Spencer Museum of Art, University of Kansas, Gift of Earl Iversen, 1978.0046.

Project in San Francisco, a loosely Buddhist-adjacent organization that started as part of a cancer institute at the University of California San Francisco several years before the emergence of AIDS. Drawing on the concept of *shanti*, a Sanskrit word meaning inner peace, the Shanti Project offered a wide array of services for people with HIV/AIDS and instituted a specific model of peer support that centered on holistic care.[4] Clearly, religion mattered in the AIDS response across the country and globally, sometimes in positive ways and other times in negative ways. What sets the heartland apart from its coastal counterparts is that on the coasts, religious-based responses were often in addition to other social service and activist efforts, whether they were state-run, nonprofit, or LGBTQ community-based programs; in the heartland, religious-based responses were not an add-on—they constituted the bulk of the AIDS response infrastructure. Within these religious responses, there is certainly a great deal to pick apart, analyze, and understand. This chapter explores why and how religion came to be so central to, and often collaborative with, the heartland AIDS response and history.

Looking more closely at the construction and deployment of the heartland white imaginary introduced in chapter 1, Christianity and morality are the lynchpins that hold the heartland white imaginary together, both

Religion 53

materially and as an imaginary formation. Religion allows for the intense shrinking of government social safety nets by offering to replace them with religious-based services. Simultaneously, Christianity provides a moralistic narrative that can easily echo the neoliberal ideals of hard work, self-sufficiency, and an innately flawed state that propels the white heartland imaginary. In this way, religion, and Christianity in particular, proved to be not only a central component of the white heartland imaginary but also a critical and material transmitter of neoliberal ideals through sermons and religious services. In the 1980s, Ronald Reagan, the rising Religious Right, and capitalists all deployed the white heartland imaginary to idealize a smaller social safety net, lower taxes, working harder, and devotion to religious institutions that echoed these financial and political aims in their religious teachings.

The narrow understanding of heartland religiosity as conservative, Protestant, and inflexible with regard to sexuality is a critical component of the heartland imaginary construct. It is a religious narrative carefully constructed and designed by the Religious Right to dovetail with conservative political aims on a larger scale and to deny the diversity of religion. It flattens, homogenizes, and erases the religious complexity and variety at play on the heartland landscape. The role of religion in the heartland AIDS response lends itself to clarifying the deployment of a heartland religion conflated with conservative Christianity while also illuminating the much broader reality of religion in the region. Several scholars have laid the groundwork for me to explore the religious diversity in the region and examine how responses to social and cultural issues vary even within a single religion in the region.[5] Thus, the heartland emerges as deeply impacted and shaped by religion. However, it is far from the ubiquitous, mythical, and homogenous conservative Protestantism that the Religious Right suggests through its conflation of religion with the white heartland imaginary.

This symbiotic relationship between political conservatism and religion in the 1980s insisted on piety, or at least a performative morality, to claim membership or feel at home in the white heartland imaginary. While a clearly defined moral code is rarely devoutly adhered to by the individual, its strong articulation through popular culture, political discourse, and commercial interests at the time armed the region with an imagined moral high ground. It is on this moral high ground that a battle over AIDS responses unfolds in the region, with some calling on the religious teachings of kindness and love, and others drawing on an urge to point out and punish the perceived moral failings of the infected. The rise of the Religious Right, which coincided with the first decade of the AIDS epidemic, is frequently and rightfully implicated in the social and political construction of the epidemic. With closer examination, we see that individual religiously affiliated hospitals and liberal congregations in many large coastal cities served as important frontline responders to the disease. However, the official stances on homosexuality and safe sex that many denominations held, not to mention the fuel for AIDS discrimination, phobia, and violence offered by the "hate the sin, not the sinner" rhetoric, rendered organized religion an overwhelmingly negative force in the AIDS epidemic.[6] A closer look at the heartland AIDS response muddies these waters and adds nuance and great complexity.

Like the heartland white imaginary, the construction/denial/reinvention of home in the region was also often entangled with religion. Religious institutions regularly served as theoretical homes, often deeply entwined with the material homes of many people, including those who became central to the regional AIDS response. Chapter 2 introduced three major groups of actors in the regional AIDS response: those who stayed in the heartland, those who moved to or within the heartland, and those who left the heartland. For many who never left the region, religious institutions, most frequently a church or youth group, proved central to their relationship with home. This played out in many ways, as some found acceptance and expansion of the home through support and validation in religious spaces while others experienced what was often their first denial of home when they were ostracized from religious spaces. For those who moved within or returned to the heartland in search of home, again, religion played a central role. Several people I interviewed spoke of myriad and unrelated chains of migration that originated from friendships and relationships in church youth groups.[7] As church groups were a common social and political anchor for communities both large and small across the region, finding a religious home was often imperative for creating a larger sense of belonging, especially for those who stood in contrast to the white heartland imaginary. Religion also played an active role in forcing some from the region, in some instances literally chasing, bullying, or shaming people away from the heartland. Here, we see religious institutions and religion itself as an extension of the material and theoretical home for both individuals and the regional AIDS response—deeply contested, denied, and reconstructed, and often at the center of community.

The power of religious institutions in relation to the AIDS response manifested in three main ways in the heartland: first, in their unmatched pre-existing infrastructure for sharing services and information; second, in their ability to coordinate, fundraise, and deploy respectability to create new AIDS responses; and third, in their ability to manifest and catalyze the widespread devotion and religious belief that permeated the populations who were either most impacted by or most responsive to HIV/AIDS in the region. While religion played a different role in this region than on the coasts, I want to be clear that religion and religious institutions did not respond in a monolithic way to the AIDS crisis. In reality, individual institutions, religious leaders, and denominations shaped their messaging around HIV/AIDS to act as a help or a cudgel to those communities most impacted by the disease, or most often some blend of both. Rarely did they only either challenge aspects of the white heartland imaginary from within the safe respectability confines of religion or use their religiosity to further entrench white heartland imaginary ideals. They most frequently molded understandings of the disease itself, those it most impacted, and the work of responding in ways that both challenged and reinforced aspects of the white heartland imaginary.

To illustrate the complex role of religion in the AIDS response and its relationship to the white heartland imaginary and concepts of home, I have chosen three specific religious organizations on which to focus in this chapter: Trinity Episcopal Church in St. Louis, DOORWAYS (a St. Louis–based nonprofit focused on housing for people with HIV/AIDS), and the Westboro Baptist Church, based in Topeka, Kansas. These three examples representing Episcopalian, interdenominational with a strong Catholic hand, and Baptist faiths provide a broad spectrum of religion-based responses to AIDS that blended home, heartland imaginary, and faith in different measures and with very different results. Discussion of some of the countless other religious organizations peppering the region appears throughout the book, especially in chapter 4, on medicine. However, these three organizations provided the richest archives, the largest impacts, and the starkest contrasts to each other in their deployments of white heartland ideals and concepts of home, making them worthy of my focus here.

Trinity, DOORWAYS, and Westboro also present some unique attributes that deserve identifying and exploring before jumping into the discussion. First of all, both Trinity and DOORWAYS call St. Louis home, and St. Louis is not just a religious city but a Catholic religious city, which makes its religious landscape quite different from other areas in the region and sets it interestingly adjacent to the white heartland imaginary. In the words of one man who moved to St. Louis from Washington, DC, mid-crisis, "For gays . . . there was this still real desire to remain in the church, versus people we knew in DC who would be like ex-Catholics."[8] With a small number of exceptions, the nearly thirty people from St. Louis I interviewed have had strong religious roots, and many continued to be active in religious communities that spanned from Catholic to Protestant to Jewish after their coming out or involvement with AIDS activism. St. Louis religious congregations proved to be important cultural, political, and social institutions regardless of one's faith or agnosticism, such that activists and congregants knew the names of liberal congregations across the religious spectrum and were fluent enough in doctrines and ethos to know how best to harness each group for an effective AIDS response. Religious groups were tied to local social services as they either administered them, legitimated them through endorsement, or funded them through congregational fundraising or charitable organizations, and often all three. Catholicism dominated this landscape, not because its subscribers far outnumber those of other religious denominations but because the city's strong and historic Catholic roots had shaped the politics and culture of the city since its founding. Westboro Baptist, though born of a form of Christianity more traditionally associated with the white heartland imaginary and ideals, is unique in the extremism and protest central to the congregation. With these caveats that make these examples exceptional, they all deploy the concepts of the white heartland imaginary and home in vastly different ways in response to the AIDS crisis, providing a sort of full spectrum on which most religious institutions in the region appear.

St. Louis, in addition to hosting two of these examples, is an important city in the heartland that deserves special attention. Consisting of St. Louis City and the surrounding St. Louis County, with the county serving as a wealthier, more suburban ancillary to the city, St. Louis has a rich history in manufacturing, transportation, and (im)migration that gives the city an industrial urban feel. Like that of many other major towns and cities in the region, St. Louis's origin story is closely tied to trade and proximity to major rivers and, eventually, railroads in its early years. However, its unique geographic situation sets it apart from its regional counterparts. Its position, perched on the banks of the Mississippi River looking across at Southern Illinois yet within proximity to both Arkansas and Tennessee, and home to its famous Gateway Arch to the West, mark the city as a crossroads of the heartland, if not the nation. While other major towns and cities in the heartland (except for Chicago, which outpaced St. Louis in this regard) were largely hubs of regional trade and business, St. Louis was decidedly an interregional hotspot.

St. Louis's proximity to rail, water, and roadways translated into economic prosperity that was tied more to manufacturing and trade than to agriculture, as in many of its regional counterparts. It remains second behind Detroit in automobile manufacturing in the United States and has strong ties not just to the industry but also to automotive history, as home to the first gas station, interstate highway, and car accident, again illustrating a sense of movement and change ingrained in the city. At the turn of the twentieth century, when St. Louis was the fourth-largest city in the country and host to both the World's Fair and the Olympics, it brimmed with Irish and German immigrants, who were followed by Italians, Greeks, Serbians, and Syrians who continue to make their marks in the neighborhoods and culture of the city today. Between the world wars, the Great Migration brought hundreds of thousands of African Americans to the city, and rich cultural additions like BBQ and the blues became synonymous with the city, even though its segregation laws made clear to Black residents the limits of its acceptance of them. By the 1950s, the population peaked at just over 800,000. However, hemmed in by the Mississippi River and the St. Louis County borders, the city couldn't expand further. This, combined with white flight and the ensuing economic plight, led to a decrease in St. Louis's population and prominence in the postwar decades.

Within the larger heartland region, St. Louis still holds the mantle of a major city. However, that doesn't translate nationally as it once did. The city itself still holds a rich history of immigrants and migration, boasting an impressive cultural infrastructure for a city of its size that hearkens back to its World's Fair and Olympic history. As today, in the 1980s, St. Louis drew younger generations from across the region looking to experience urban living, a phenomenon that grew more popular as the economic policies of the 1980s made rural life more economically challenging for many. In short, St. Louis was and is among the brightest of jewels in the crown of heartland cities, and the concept of the white heartland imaginary sometimes chafed against its metropolitan undercurrents. However, for the bulk of St. Louisans, surrounding Missourians, and certainly the crafters of the heartland imaginary, St. Louis still fell comfortably within the confines of the white heartland imaginary.

Trinity Episcopal Church

If the three examples offered here create a sort of spectrum of religious responses, Trinity Episcopal Church would land on the far left of the spectrum, as it deployed its respectability as a religious institution to push against the exclusions of the white heartland imaginary, to broaden access to home, and to build an AIDS response that destigmatized and welcomed those infected. Even with Episcopalians' historic liberal attitudes toward gender and sexuality (certainly in comparison to Roman Catholic dogma), Trinity often took this to new heights. Trinity has proven to be unusually safe for and welcoming to LGBTQ community members (but not exclusively them) since the 1950s, carefully and adroitly navigating a local topography fraught with racial tension, sexuality politics, and respectability politics in St. Louis. Located within a block of Delmar Avenue, the racial dividing line of St. Louis, and at the northern tip of the Central West End, a neighborhood long associated with the city's LGBTQ residents, Trinity deployed two tactics to engage with the surrounding community, including members of the LGBTQ community, without proselytizing overtly. One was to hold special events at Trinity designed to attract new community members into the church. The "Jazz Mass" in January 1963 epitomized this tactic, with its full band, youth choir, invitations to neighborhood residents, and even a guest preacher who commented to the national religious publication *Now* that "[priest] Morely and I are convinced that many people will come to this service out of curiosity who might otherwise never darken the doorway of Trinity Church."[9] The second approach involved Trinity reaching beyond the church walls, going out into spaces that attracted a "bohemian" (that is, gay) crowd. As Ian Darnell explains, "In 1964, a coalition of St. Louis churches opened a coffeehouse called the Exit . . . a few blocks from Trinity . . . near a number of gay bars and cafés." Open at night, staffed by volunteers from area churches, and hosting poetry readings and folk music performances, the Exit attracted "hordes" of patrons, including many of the neighborhood's "Bohemian residents," according to *Now*.[10] By throwing its doors open intentionally to the diversity in the Central West End and going out into the community, Trinity sought to make clear to all in the Central West End that it hoped to serve everyone, that it could be a home to all. It both relied on and stretched the limits of its assumed respectability as a local church. On the one hand, by growing its work and presence beyond both the physical and spiritual areas of the church, it blurred the role of the church and the "place" for religion. On the other hand, simultaneously, it also expanded the meaning of respectable churchgoers in the larger community to include many who had been typically denied by the white heartland imaginary, religious hardliners, and homophobia.

Trinity solidified its role as a left-leaning activist church repeatedly over the late twentieth century while carefully maintaining its legitimacy as a site of respectability and religious devotion. As other area churches responded to the white flight of the immediate post–World War II years by moving to the suburbs, the Trinity congregation held a vote in 1953 and opted to stay in their urban setting, declaring that its calling was to meet the needs and challenges of the changing neighborhood. Within months of the April 1969 founding of the Mandrake Society, St. Louis's first homophile organization, Trinity permanently became its meeting place, offering refuge to Mandrake members as the church sought to "equalize the state and position of the homosexual with the status and position of the heterosexual."[11] The eighteen dues-paying members met twice a month at the church throughout the autumn of 1969.[12] Plainclothes police officers from the St. Louis Police Department's vice division waited outside a Central West End gay bar a few blocks from both Trinity and the site of the Exit coffeehouse shortly after midnight on November 1 that year. As the Halloween drag ball inside began to disperse, the officers arrested a group of nine men clad in wigs, jewelry, heels, and evening gowns, for violating the city's anti-masquerading ordinance. Members of the Mandrake Society, using its phone tree in place for just such an occasion, raised the alarm and called for an immediate protest. By 3:00 A.M. on November 1, 1969, nearly two dozen protesters stood outside the St. Louis police headquarters demanding the men's release. The ACLU (American Civil Liberties Union) refused to take the case, but the Mandrake Society helped finance the men's defense until the judge dismissed the charges.[13] The arrests and resulting protest solidified Trinity's role as the birthplace of the St. Louis gay rights struggle as the regularly scheduled November 1969 Mandrake Society meeting drew 150 people to Trinity. One new attendee was an owner of a gay coffeehouse "concerned about the welfare of some of her boys . . . who had been arrested."[14] By January, the Mandrake Society had over 100 dues-paying members who attended meetings, and the surrounding community saw the church as a beacon: "Trinity accepts people for what they are."[15] It paid to get this message across by advertising in the newsletter of the Mandrake Society, the first of its kind in the city. The newsletter, available in bars and gay businesses in the Central West End and beyond, provided Trinity with the opportunity not only to welcome and support gay parishioners and community members but also to grow Trinity's reputation as a welcoming and inclusive congregation and meeting place for members of the LGBTQ communities. The advertisement speaks directly to this message: "All people, including each of you, are invited to attend all services in this historic Anglo-Catholic parish church whose special mission is to serve the entire community."[16] This advertising, along with the housing of the Mandrake Society, the community outreach programs, and the direct engagement of gay activists by members of the ministry team, attracted gay men and lesbians to Trinity in numbers that grew steadily. These actions also set Trinity apart from any other religious institution in the St. Louis area during the late 1960s and 1970s and allowed it to weave together its spiritual calling with social and political movements. In short, it stretched the notion of religious home as well as the role of the church itself in the community. In the words of one community member, "One must look to Trinity Episcopal Church at Euclid and Washington, a cornerstone of the religious community in that area, as a factor in fostering the rise of a Gay ghetto."[17]

Trinity made the practice of this dogma quotidian, not just in moments of strife, stress, or attack. Gays and lesbians from the surrounding neighborhood and city joined the choir, served on the Trinity lay leadership board, and expanded the church's outreach efforts further.[18] Before the end of the decade, Trinity also became home to the St. Louis chapter of the Gay Liberation Front, which included three Trinity congregants, a gay episcopal group called Integrity, a gay youth group named Youth of America, and even a group for gay Catholics.[19] Whether they were members of the Trinity congregation or not, politically active gays and lesbians of St. Louis knew they were welcome at Trinity and that the church provided a haven for LGBTQ people as well as a launching pad for many of the city's LGBT services and organizations in the 1970s. Trinity very intentionally provided a home, especially for those whose relationship to home was complicated by sexuality.

However, Trinity didn't just ask for a commitment to the church from its gay parishioners; it also asked the full congregation to engage with and commit to spiritual explorations of sexuality. In a racially and sexually diverse congregation, not to mention one affiliated with a religion that remained highly critical of homosexuality throughout this period, creating opportunities for dialogue and reflection became a hallmark of the parish. Darnell explains that the priest at the time, "[Bill] Chapman, was very conscious of Trinity's unusual identity as a congregation that was both racially mixed and welcoming to gays, and he encouraged parishioners to think through how this fit into their lived experience of faith." During Lent in 1976, for example, he led a weekly series of discussions of "Christian Perspectives" on the following topics: "Sexuality and Vocation," "Sexuality and Ordination," "Race and Identity," "Race and Power," and "Race and Community."[20]

Engaging in these sometimes difficult and spiritually fraught conversations set the Trinity congregation apart, as it clearly tried to push the meanings of home, respectability, and even the heartland to new heights. Through these conversations and efforts, Trinity undermined the white heartland imaginary as a place in which religion worked to reinforce heteronormativity, homophobia, whiteness, and independence. In short, the church used the cover of respectability to subvert the white heartland imaginary ideals without losing credibility. While the white heartland imaginary sought to diminish access to home and belonging for those who contradicted the carefully crafted idealized white heartland citizen, Trinity's activity expanded the walls of both the physical and theoretical notions of home to be more inclusive. The tactic of deploying respectability and harnessing the protective power of straight allies by way of religion was not unique to Trinity or even to the heartland region. Hanhardt's *Safe Space* and J. H. Miller's work exploring the San Francisco Council on Religion and the Homosexual (CRH) outline the evolution and important deployments of this tactic, demonstrating that religion and LGBTQ history are deeply intertwined, and not always in negative ways.[21] Just as the CRH sought to ameliorate the violence and mistreatment of homosexuals in the 1960s by fostering dialogue with the religious communities in San Francisco, so too did Trinity Episcopal Church in St. Louis in the 1970s. When San Francisco police raided a CRH meeting, religious leaders and community members offered themselves as buffers to police harassment of homosexual members of the group.[22] While Trinity was never raided, it certainly positioned itself in very similar ways and reflected the larger history of the relationship between homophile and gay liberationist activism and religion.[23]

When AIDS first emerged in 1981, St. Louis's response was tempered by its more religiously and politically conservative landscape as well as the comparatively meager gay service infrastructure, and Trinity found its calling renewed. Again, Trinity proved to be a trailblazer in the first years of the epidemic as a religious organization not exclusively for gay parishioners (MCC remained the only specifically LGBTQ church) that quickly responded to the AIDS crisis. As it had with the gay political groups of the 1970s, Trinity provided support during the AIDS crisis in the gay community by offering its physical space. In 1984, a small group including Daniel Flier, John Allen, and other gay activists and people with AIDS founded the St. Louis Effort for AIDS, the city's first AIDS-related social service organization. Initial meetings and operations were held in a room above a gay bar in the Central West End but later moved into the North Parish Hall of Trinity Episcopal Church. While housed in Trinity, St. Louis Effort for AIDS officially incorporated and secured nonprofit status in late 1985 with a modest $6,000 budget mostly raised by asking friends for donations at dinner parties held by the founders.[24] St. Louis Effort for AIDS provided (and continues to provide) a broad range of services, from up-to-date information about the disease and its treatments and support groups for people with AIDS and those around them to projects connecting people with AIDS with food aid, housing, pet care, buddy systems, and government programs. Trinity also played host to the Privacy Right Education Project (PREP), which was founded in 1986 after the *Bowers v. Hardwick* Supreme Court decision upheld the laws forbidding sodomy in Georgia.[25] This organization, which went on to become PROMO (Promoting Missouri), the statewide organization advocating for LGBTQ equality, initially advocated for several causes that related to privacy rights, including the rights of people with AIDS to confidentiality from their doctors, as the public reporting of one's HIV-positive status frequently led to job loss, home eviction, and other forms of discrimination.[26] Trinity also occasionally provided space to the short-lived St. Louis ACT UP chapter and partnered with the Metropolitan St. Louis AIDS Program through its food ministry to provide healthy food to people living with AIDS.[27]

In addition to offering meeting space and forms of financial support like buying ads in newsletters to the main AIDS social service and political agencies in the city, "Trinity Episcopal Church was an early haven for people with AIDS."[28] A handful of congregants became HIV-positive in the 1980s, and the parish organized to care for them as they became weaker and died. People with AIDS also joined the Trinity congregation as a result of its openness and dedication to those living with the disease.[29] In 1986, Rev. Charles Bewick was forced to leave both his position and his congregation in another local parish after his HIV-positive status became known. Trinity became his new spiritual home, inviting him to occasionally preach when his health allowed. Church clergy and volunteers from the congregation nursed him as he experienced numerous near-fatal illnesses until he succumbed to AIDS in 1989. That year, a "hearty handful of Trinitarians" marched in the Pride parade with a banner honoring Rev. Bewick, and an artwork commemorating Rev. Bewick still hangs in the Trinity Episcopal Church today, a testament to the congregation's dedication and pride in serving those most in need amid the AIDS crisis.[30] In the late 1980s, as AIDS-related deaths in St. Louis began to accelerate, Trinity faced one of the grim realities of both the disease and the stigma that came with it as individuals who "were pushed away from their families and home churches" needed burials. "In April of 1989, Chapman [the reverend at Trinity] reported to the vestry that burials of people not members of Trinity, especially victims of AIDS 'isolated from their own churches,' would be performed."[31]

Trinity also worked beyond the boundaries of the church walls to battle the stigma of AIDS. "In 1986, the Very Rev. Michael Allen, Dean, Christ Church Cathedral, asked Trinity to co-sponsor an AIDS workshop for the Diocese," and on November 9 of that year, the church joined with the national church to remember AIDS victims.[32] As the epidemic's size and scope came into clearer focus in the late 1980s, Trinity provided a rallying cry to other area churches to join the fight, evidenced by Rev. Chapman joining with Trinity member Dr. George Tucker in January 1988 to present "AIDS and the Churches" at Emmanuel Episcopal Church in Webster Groves. Chapman also used the power of his position and reputation in the community to encourage media coverage of the epidemic that was less fear-driven and homophobic, writing letters to news outlets about their coverage.[33] In these efforts, Trinity responded to the AIDS crisis with compassion and love, providing a refuge for people with AIDS and undertaking and nurturing efforts to make St. Louis a kinder and safer place to be a person with AIDS. In whatever way it could imagine, Trinity attempted to broaden understandings of home and heartland rather than bend to a more "respectable footing" that might have been more widely accepted by the larger heartland.

DOORWAYS

On the spectrum of the relationship between religion and white heartland ideals in the AIDS response, DOORWAYS lands in the middle, meaning that it built a strong and collaborative AIDS response but often did so by deploying aspects of the white heartland imaginary and constructions of home strategically and in service to its own ends. The lack of healthy and multifaceted political and social service infrastructure within the region's most impacted communities—in part a result of a relatively small out gay population and largely segregated and ignored communities of color—demanded a politically collaborative response to the epidemic that relied on groups not often thought of as allies. Thus, the need for buy-in from religious institutions and traditionally more conservative community stakeholders shaped the early AIDS response in the heartland. The creation and evolution of DOORWAYS, a housing organization for people with HIV/AIDS in St. Louis, provides a window into the mechanics of the epidemic's political framing to address the crisis in the political landscape of the region—a framework that resonated throughout the region and reverberated back into the national lesbian, gay, and bisexual political agenda of the 1980s, 1990s, and 2000s.

On the heartland landscape, organizations such as DOORWAYS emerged as some of the most transformational sites of activism as they provided desperately needed services while simultaneously challenging people largely unaffected by the HIV/AIDS epidemic to engage with the epidemic morally, spiritually, and financially. To procure widespread support, DOORWAYS bartered in respectability politics, making those in need "worthy" and "appealing to donors" by foregrounding particular stories of AIDS and deemphasizing others. Examining the role of religion in DOORWAYS provides an insightful analysis of how some religious institutions leveraged their respectability to respond to the AIDS crisis, to push against and sometimes reinforce the cruelest effects of the white heartland imaginary and provide at least a physical home to those in need. The case of DOORWAYS enables a clear view of the importance of religion, religious communities, and interdenominational alliances in the regional response. It also provides a sharp contrast to the way that religious institutions factor into the AIDS history of the coasts.

Archbishop of St. Louis John L. May is nearly universally credited with mainstreaming St. Louis's AIDS response. Appointed archbishop in 1980 by Pope John Paul II, May quickly became known as a bridge builder and a firm believer in both ecumenism and interfaith collaboration around social issues. He regularly said, "I will pray with anyone," and he proved it when the lesbian and gay Catholic group Dignity invited him to join them in prayer in the first few years of his tenure. The move was a careful navigation of a deeply contested issue within the Catholic Church, which forbade administering communion to homosexuals, which made clear May's devotion to following Vatican policies and his desire to bridge divisions with controversial groups.[34] This measured approach in every aspect of his ministry ultimately led to his 1986 election to a three-year term as the president of the National Conference of Catholic Bishops. These three years would place the Catholic Church in the crosshairs of AIDS activists, and May's role is both surprising and understudied in the larger literature on this period. In his role as president, May oversaw the penning (by another heartland bishop from Chicago) and approval of a 1987 statement on AIDS titled *The Many Faces of AIDS: A Gospel Response*, which, in its thirty pages, indicated qualified support for the use of and education about condoms. To be clear, this support was limited in many ways and appeared only after restatement of the Church's stance against homosexuality, sex outside of marriage, and many other issues, which many AIDS activists and LGBT people found discriminatory:

> Because we live in a pluralistic society, we acknowledge that some will not agree with our understanding of human sexuality. We recognize that public educational programs addressed to a wide audience will reflect the fact that some people will not act as they can and should; that they will not refrain from the type of sexual or drug abuse behavior

that can transmit AIDS. In such situations, educational efforts, if grounded in the broader moral vision outlined above, *could include accurate information about prophylactic devices* or other practices proposed by some medical experts as potential means of preventing AIDS. *We are not promoting the use of prophylactics*, but merely providing information that is part of the factual picture. Such a factual presentation should indicate that abstinence outside of marriage and fidelity within marriage as well as the avoidance of intravenous drug abuse are the only morally correct and medically sure ways to prevent the spread of AIDS. So-called safe sex practices are at best only partially effective. They do not take into account either the real values that are at stake or the fundamental good of the human person. (emphasis added)[35]

While AIDS activists found much to be frustrated with in this shaming of sexual practices outside heterosexual monogamy (as well as several other issues in the statement and in the general teachings of the Catholic Church), the critique that proved the most consequential in the larger AIDS narrative came from one of the most conservative cardinals in the conference. Cardinal O'Connor of New York, who had not attended the conference meeting where the statement originated, corresponded with May about what he believed were the errors in this policy, made public excerpts of May's response, declared the policy in abeyance, and garnered support from conservative bishops around the country to nullify the policy.[36] O'Connor did his best to undermine and overturn the policy about prophylactics before it could be implemented. O'Connor's vocal dissent placed him at the center of several ACT UP actions in New York, including the die-in at St. Patrick's Cathedral in New York City that resulted in dozens of arrests and continues to (problematically) epitomize the role of religion in the coastal AIDS narrative.[37] However, May stood by the statement, issuing additional statements reiterating the policy, which had been approved by vote and gone through all the proper channels.

As the National Conference of Catholic Bishops became increasingly divided over the issue, with bishops siding with either O'Connor or May, May agreed to take the issue up at the following year's meeting.[38] However, the recording of the proceedings suggests May placed the item near the end of the meeting's agenda, ensuring it didn't get taken up in 1988.[39] Finally, as May's term came to a close at the 1989 meeting of the National Conference of Catholic Bishops, O'Connor had garnered enough support for a newly drafted and much more conservative statement, titled *Called to Compassion and Responsibility*, which, among other shifts to the right, strongly condemned the use of or education about prophylactics of any kind.[40] The measure passed within days of the end of May's term, solidifying the Catholic Church's position as a nemesis of AIDS activists on the national stage and certainly in cities like New York and Boston that had the most conservative church leadership.

Those tumultuous and divisive years of May's leadership of the National Conference of Catholic Bishops stood in stark contrast to May's concomitant time as the archbishop of St. Louis. Standing by the initial statement's stance on teaching about prophylactics, May focused his attention locally on many of the larger issues the statement enumerated as contributing to the pandemic, such as poverty, inequality, access to healthcare, and the public's fear of the infected. Consequently, St. Louisans responded to the Catholic Church differently than their counterparts in New York City. In fact, the Catholic archbishop of St. Louis, John May, is frequently referred to as "the Spiritual parent of DOORWAYS."[41] He instigated an interdenominational working group, including religious leaders from the biggest religious congregations in the city (such as Rabbi Ruben from Temple Israel and Rev. Michael Allen from Christ Church Cathedral), community activists, and representatives from the city's main AIDS service organizations. In these meetings, housing emerged as the most obvious and basic roadblock for health services, a concept that fueled the interdenominational funding and volunteering commitment. All the religious leaders both present and represented in those meetings echoed this notion of housing as essential to health in their statements to their congregants and to other liberal religious leaders in the city. Michael Allen, a liberal Episcopal priest with Christ Church Cathedral (the main cathedral for St. Louis) "was masterful . . . at tapping his wealthy and connected parishioners, particularly in the business community [to fundraise for DOORWAYS]. He said in his pulpit that St. Louis has AIDS, and we have AIDS, Christ Church has AIDS."[42] It became a cause célèbre among liberal churches and temples, evidenced by the funds raised and volunteers regularly recruited over the next several years.

To be clear, housing was a need for people with HIV/AIDS, but it was also an almost uniquely palatable issue for religious-based coalitions to rally behind. For one thing, the idea of creating a home resonates across many religions, whether it evokes the Jews longing for Israel, Joseph and Mary settling for a manger, or the central analogy of houses of worship as extensions of home for parishioners. Home has a great deal of religious symbolism, both metaphorically and materially. And if we move beyond the religious realm, we see that housing also ticks many boxes with respect to the white heartland imaginary. Providing those in need with a home opens the pathways to self-sufficiency and creates a place where one can be sick without drawing on the services of the state. It strikes a balance between relying on the nuclear family (which often was not an option) and relying solely on state services for care. Housing also allows for privacy for individuals, where they can better conceal how they do not conform to white heartland ideals. By focusing on the physical spaces, religious institutions could overlook and simultaneously erase the actions most associated with the spread of AIDS, including drug use, homosexual sex, and sex outside of marriage. Housing was and is a critical need, but it is also easily and entirely divorced from sexuality and drug use, making it the perfect issue for a religious collaboration in the heartland.

With housing the sick and needy downplaying homosexuality, condoms, and drug use, liberal religious congregations and individuals of different faiths threw their full support behind DOORWAYS in multiple ways. Fundraising ranged from parishioners passing the basket during weekly services to business leaders with religious ties sponsoring event sponsorships, and from organizations providing generous start-up funding (for example, $75,000 from the Jewish Foundation) to religious foundations taking on quarterly obligations.[43] In the early years, Catholic Charities was donating "something like $50,000" quarterly.[44] There was also evidence of "God on the ground" with congregants volunteering and with individuals with strong religious ties running DOORWAYS. The first executive director of DOORWAYS was an ex-nun named Lynn Cooper, who "could talk anybody into anything" and who partnered with an active nun, Sister Betty, an administrator at a local Catholic hospital, to bring DOORWAYS to life.[45] Both women were "tough" people "you didn't say no to" but also "incredibly kind."[46] Sister Betty used her power as a hospital administrator to secure the city's first designated hospital beds for AIDS patients, and when nurses and doctors balked at her decision, she fired them. She also helped Cooper identify a convent in the city that had unused living quarters and instigated negotiations for their use as DOORWAYS's first living spaces for people with AIDS.[47] The hospital beds, convent quarters, and rent subsidy program provided the foundation on which DOORWAYS could be built. As word spread about the DOORWAYS mission, through congregations and announcements in weekly religious bulletins, property owners began to donate properties or sought rental partnerships with DOORWAYS.[48] The organization offered more than altruistic incentives for business-minded property owners, as DOORWAYS "always paid on time" from its religiously funded bank accounts, and initially (before becoming more discerning), it offered unscrupulous property owners opportunities to off-load dilapidated buildings for a tax break.[49] Seemingly, in St. Louis and in other cities that copied the DOORWAYS model, religious associations opened many doors that otherwise would have been closed.

As women, and specifically women of color, accounted for increasing numbers of new HIV/AIDS infections in the city, DOORWAYS further disassociated itself from homosexuality. By centering women rather than gay men in the DOORWAYS mission and the AIDS crisis more generally, DOORWAYS increased the palatability of its work to its religious stakeholders, particularly Black pastors. Although Archbishop May's interdenominational working group and many of the nonprofits that also made up the St. Louis AIDS response had repeatedly extended invitations to numerous Black pastors, they proved unwilling to openly engage, at least initially.[50] Their reluctance appears to have been driven partly by the connection between AIDS and homosexuality, but it was also the response required by the Black respectability politics at work within the highly segregated city of St. Louis. Too often, scholars associate Black churches with homophobia without digging deeper to reveal the political enactment of respectability and rebuttal of negative sexual stereotypes that all but necessitate the shunning of the sexual practices or drug use behind the AIDS epidemic. Works by Cathy Cohen, Daniel Royles, Darius Bost, and others tease out and provide nuanced insight into this political conundrum.[51] However, as the impact of AIDS on communities of Black women became more pronounced and stood outside the bounds of gay and/or intravenous drug-using populations, Black churches became more engaged in the St. Louis AIDS response, often through the carefully sanitized work of DOORWAYS. All religious stakeholders in DOORWAYS, including Black churches, mobilized the innocent (and respectable) victim narratives offered by mothers and women infected with the disease to raise funds, awareness, and sympathy among their congregants.[52] DOORWAYS shifted its vision from "country club/fraternity house(s)" for gay men with AIDS to family-friendly housing and housing for all low-income people with AIDS. By focusing on poverty and de-emphasizing people of color and homosexuality, DOORWAYS redeployed certain aspects of the white heartland imaginary to ultimately build housing for a much more diverse set of characters.

In this way, DOORWAYS, more than any other AIDS service organization in St. Louis, successfully bridged the highly segregated St. Louis landscape with buildings and apartments located all over the city, integrated living spaces in predominantly white or Black neighborhoods, and invested stakeholders spanning the religious and racial spectrums. Against the backdrop of infected women, Black pastors and neighborhood leaders welcomed DOORWAYS with open arms, inviting the organization to build and rent numerous housing developments, including the Mama Nyumba and Kaya Malaika buildings designed specifically for mothers and children—two of just a few of their kind in the nation.[53] Meanwhile, the organization also continued to provide outreach and services for gay men and those infected through intravenous drug use. This somewhat clandestine and collaborative relationship between the straight Black community and gay communities played out beyond the AIDS crisis in the city.[54] When Mary Ross, the city alderman and former chairwoman of the Black caucus, introduced and pushed through a civil rights ordinance in 1992 that included some of the strongest protections for gays and lesbians in the country, she did so by highlighting the creation of a civil rights commission with investigative and disciplinary power and downplaying the inclusion of gay rights.[55] In an interview with the *New York Times* several weeks after passage of the ordinance, Ross explained, "I think we covered, hopefully, everybody in this legislation who could possibly be discriminated against in one manner or another, and that is the intent. It is not a gay-rights thing."[56] As a result, St. Louis's protections for gays and lesbians passed unanimously and without incident, while by contrast, the Kansas City "gay" ordinance spearheaded by local gay and lesbian activists took years of protracted debate and protests.[57]

While the religiously inspired sanitizing politics deployed by DOORWAYS opened many, well, doorways, it darkened others. For DOORWAYS, fundraising in the larger community, away from the official churches, was conscientiously tailored to be appropriate for the nuns and ex-nuns associated with the organization.[58] This is just one example of how such firm ties with religion had a comparatively conservatizing effect on the gay community's response to AIDS. Looking beyond DOORWAYS, we can see the religious influence in the broader St. Louis AIDS response in other ways—specifically, the power of the closet. Though St. Louis has a rich LGBTQ history, nearly all of my interviewees point to the closet as the greatest impediment to a more robust AIDS response.[59] One said, "The gays that were here in St. Louis at that time were much more closeted. . . . Some of it had to do with religion, some of it had to do with, um, they were from here, and their families were still here."[60] Gay chain migration in St. Louis—in which gay men built on friendships forged in small rural and often evangelical congregations to gain entry into gay networks and spaces in St. Louis, where older youths or youth ministers had moved and come out—was a shared experience among many who migrated to the city. These homegrown friendships served as both a gateway and a checkpoint, meaning that new arrivals had a built-in community that not only connected them to gay spaces and people but also could potentially report on them back home.[61] Certainly, stories of the closet appear in coastal histories of AIDS too, but St. Louis, though one of the twenty most populous cities in the country in the early 1980s and the largest in the state at the time, operated very much as a small town. Numerous interview subjects commented on the city's insular nature, explaining that people commonly mentioned where they went to high school in their initial introductions and that often, knowledge of (or even relationships with) their extended family members preceded them.

Concerning the AIDS epidemic, this ethos played out in countless ways, regardless of how "out" an individual was: families learned of their sons' sexuality and HIV/AIDS infection in the same breath in hospital waiting rooms; gay men limited their involvement with gay politics to avoid word getting back to their families; and safe-sex workshops modeled on those in coastal cities toned it down for the St. Louis crowd.[62] Commenting on how St. Louis was more conservative about sex than other big cities he had lived in and visited, one DOORWAYS member recalled, "In San Francisco, when they did [a safe-sex workshop called] Hot, Healthy, and Horny, they did the education training and then would have a safe-sex party. Well, the safe-sex party would never work in St. Louis. . . . [In] St. Louis you could talk about it, but you can't get together and do it."[63] The religiosity of the city, deeply tied to the white heartland imaginary, translated into a prudishness in public, even within gay spaces and culture. The religious attempts to erase sexuality from AIDS discussions in ways that inherently placed blame and shame on certain sexualities and acts reinforced the St. Louis gay community's assumption that "you weren't gonna get AIDS if you weren't out there every night having sex with ten people . . . and only people that did that would ever get AIDS."[64] This, in turn, fueled AIDS discrimination within the gay communities of St. Louis and associated it with the judgment-laden notion of promiscuity that operated both in gay communities and in conservative political rhetoric. This conservatism was informed by the larger political landscape of the city and region, the looming power of the white heartland imaginary. Not acting with discretion could and did have real consequences, particularly around AIDS. When word got out to the larger St. Louis community that a local AIDS service organization specifically for the Black community had invited a famous gay stripper and porn actor to an event, the resulting negative press and funding recoil shuttered the organization within months.[65]

Though the success and exponential growth of DOORWAYS speak to an acceptance of people with AIDS and the religious-infused mission to help them, simply associating religion with the act of housing people with AIDS did not defuse the fear and bigotry roused by the illness. There is an equal number of examples of AIDS phobia and homophobia that housing people with AIDS inspired. Initially, residents living near potential DOORWAYS buildings or rentals had a "not in my backyard" response. Even as recently as 2018, the organization encountered a repairman who refused to do work on a building when he learned that it housed AIDS patients.[66] When an order of nuns wanted to rent a portion of their convent at a discounted rate to DOORWAYS in 1988, an adjacent hospital brought the deal to a halt because "it did not want people [with AIDS] coming into their emergency room without insurance."[67] Equally importantly, if perhaps obviously, the religious responses to AIDS in St. Louis and the heartland more generally were far from monolithic and certainly not universally positive.

The DOORWAYS response deployed respectability and bowed to other aspects of the heartland white imaginary out of necessity, relying on collaborations with religious groups because without those partnerships, the response would have been meager and anemic, if not entirely impossible. Though gay culture in the city was vibrant and multifaceted, it simply did not have the capacity or the preexisting foundations for the creation of multiple social service agencies and the fundraising that the epidemic required, which materialized in places like New York, Los Angeles, and San Francisco. In short, partnering with religious organizations and using religious infrastructure to mobilize an AIDS response grew from practicality. Two activists explained that "St. Louis was a hard nut to crack. . . . Making them say the word 'AIDS,' making them admit they had a gay son . . . it's pretty conservative."[68] One founding board member of DOORWAYS remarked that "people were more politically conservative here. . . . St. Louis is known for being more conservative in their money, their banks, their investing, the medicine here is more conservative. The joke is that St. Louis was founded by the people who were not risk takers and not willing to go the rest of the way out west, so they stayed here."[69] Religion is a central part of this conservative landscape, even the more liberal pockets of it, and that conservatism lay at the center of the heartland white imaginary as it was deployed by various conservative power nodes in the 1980s.

However, there is also the reality of religion catalyzing congregations and business elites to provide housing to people with AIDS and congregants becoming central figures in the city's AIDS organizations. One observant Jewish woman, along with her husband, became a strident AIDS activist and critical volunteer at several St. Louis AIDS organizations after her son's death from AIDS in 1987. She remembered a moment working a hotline with another frequent volunteer when "we got the giggles because here I was, a nice Jewish matron from the West County, and here she was, this nice Catholic lady [Sister Margaret] from St. Louis City, and we're telling all these young people how to have safe sex! Can you imagine!?"[70] From this vantage point, the role of religion-driven AIDS response in subverting the white heartland imaginary was just as complex as the way it strategically drew on the often-harmful trappings of respectability and morality, aspects of the white heartland imaginary, and the meaning of home to rally support for AIDS action.

This strategy of leaning heavily on respectability and other aspects of the white heartland imaginary to manifest compassion and action for those most impacted by AIDS, which was perfected in the heartland AIDS response, became a hallmark of the local and national political agendas for numerous minority groups throughout the closing decades of the twentieth century. While this approach blurred and rearticulated white heartland ideals in interesting ways, it simultaneously made more rigid the boundaries of home. Those included in the slightly expanded heartland imaginary gained some access to home while those who remained denied were doubly so, first by the original white heartland imaginary and again even by those working to expand that landscape.

Westboro

Of these three examples, Westboro Baptist Church is the most likely to have had its reputation precede it, as it became a national example of religion-infused homophobia and AIDS phobia in the 1980s, 1990s, and even still today. On the spectrum of religion-based AIDS responses in the heartland region, Westboro anchors the far right, drawing heavily on the most rigid interpretations of the white heartland imaginary and religious texts to actively repel AIDS activists from the region and dismantle AIDS-related services and claims to home for those most impacted by the epidemic. Due to the national notoriety and long-standing national news coverage of Westboro, my description of the church and its activities will be rather brief before I pivot to an analysis of how the white heartland imaginary and concepts of home were tools utilized effectively by Westboro preacher Fred Phelps and his followers.

Fred Phelps founded the Westboro Baptist Church in Topeka, Kansas, in 1955, and he quickly became known for lambasting and vitriolic sermons, harsh even by the primary Baptist standards in which God takes on a vengeful and angry demeanor. A trained lawyer who fought against Jim Crow in Topeka in the 1960s, he turned in the 1980s from dismantling structural racism to applying his righteousness and zeal to saving society from what he saw as the ravages of homosexuality.[71] For him and his followers, both causes were religious imperatives tantamount to saving the United States from moral corruption. His fight for the soul of America would also result in his attacking the US military—the thinking being that those who fought for a United States that allowed homosexuality were condoning homosexuality. Other enemies of the Phelps congregation included Jews, Muslims, and many Christian denominations, again because they tolerated behavior Phelps found immoral, or because they were seen as violent threats to Westboro's primitive Baptist biblical interpretation.

Starting in 1989, Phelps led regular traveling protests across the country as part of the mission and work of the church. Multicolored signs reading "GOD HATES FAGS," "AMERICA HATES FAGS," "FAG TROOPS," and "MOURN FOR YOUR SINS" became well-known hallmarks of the Westboro protests, in addition to placards with anti-Semitic and anti-Muslim sentiments. But it was the use of the protest itself, particularly funeral protests, that set Westboro Baptist Church apart from other congregations, even those that embraced a more militant approach like that of Randall Terry, the founder of Operation Rescue and the firebrand of the anti-abortion movement, who also hailed from Kansas. Funeral protests became mass media events, drawing not only the press but also often huge counterprotests. During the church's height of both activity and fame in the 1990s, Westboro Baptist members would protest at several funerals every week across the country, as well as at Pride events and legislative meetings of nearly any type, at almost any level of government.[72]

They gained national notoriety, especially when they began protesting at military funerals. While protesting at the funerals of people who had AIDS and were openly gay could be directly tied to the church's homophobic and AIDS-phobic beliefs, the decision to protest military funerals was a bit more convoluted. Phelps's rationale for protesting at military funerals was twofold: first, war was a sign of God's anger at the failings of humanity (specifically around acceptance of homosexuality, Judaism, and Islam), so protesting against those who had fought and died in war was a way to underline those failings that had led to war in the first place; and second, soldiers' defense of a United States that accepted homosexuals, Jews, and Muslims was tantamount to the soldiers themselves being gay, Jewish, or Muslim, and it not only offended God but besmirched his interpretation of the United States.

Phelps deeply intertwined religion and nationalism, and, in turn, linked nationalism with whiteness, heterosexuality, hard work, independence, and a preference for self-sufficiency over state-run entitlements. In short, Phelps's church idealized a strict interpretation of the white heartland imaginary. In addition to subscribing to white heartland ideals, the Westboro Baptist Church also denied access to home in a variety of ways. Perhaps most obviously, by picketing at the literal final resting place for many, the protesters sought to deny access to a peaceful home in the material world, the spiritual world, and the discursive world. Phelps also directed his pickets at legislative meetings that were considering providing legal protection to people with AIDS, including rights to material homes in the form of housing protections. Although the city council of largely Catholic St. Louis did approve a wide-ranging civil rights bill that included gays and lesbians and people with AIDS as well as a wide array of other minoritized groups (with very little fanfare or blowback), Westboro Baptist made passing a much narrower and weaker set of protections a years-long battle in Kansas City. Public comment periods became overrun with AIDS activists on one side and Westboro Baptist parishioners on the other. Passing housing protections for people with AIDS in Kansas City took over three years of effort.[73] And Kansas City was only one of many towns and cities across the region that experienced a fever-pitch battle from Phelps as they considered how to respond to the HIV/AIDS crisis. Not surprisingly, Westboro Baptist congregants became the primary adversaries in numerous LGBTQ-related and AIDS-related issues, and they continue to be so today.[74] In each of these protests, Westboro Church members waged war over who belonged and who could call the area home without inciting God's wrath. Even within the church itself, the concept of home was wielded as a bartering chip and weapon. At the heart of the Westboro congregation was Phelps's large biological family and extended family. As his children grew up, several left the church and cut ties with their father and the larger family, and thus lost their homes in many forms. Of note, one of his thirteen children left the church to become an LGBTQ advocate and activist, as have many of his grandchildren.[75]

While Phelps deployed white heartland ideals and concepts of home in an attempt to restrict access to the heartland for people with AIDS and others he deemed outside the ideal, his actions often had the opposite effect. Kansas activist Jay Johnson explained, "Phelps, in many ways, made it easier. In the moment, he definitely made it more difficult. But in the general climate, he made it easier because then people, when they were feeling more homophobic or frightened or whatever or wanting to go evangelical, they would see the Phelps and go, 'I don't look like that, do I? Yikes!'"[76] Westboro also animated a truly unique and motley constellation of counterprotesters almost everywhere they appeared. Military veteran biker gangs would coordinate with drag queens, who would dress like angels with huge wings to shield funeral attendees from the sight of Westboro protesters. LGBTQ counterprotesters also often joined in, so counterprotesters often outnumbered the Westboro Baptist contingent.

While funerals, legislative sessions, and similarly quotidian activities sparked the protests and counterprotests that embodied a fight over the role of religion, the soul of the heartland, and the meaning of home, particularly for those impacted by AIDS (or implicated in its acceptance, in the case of military personnel). In this way, Westboro Baptist Church's role in the HIV/AIDS response in the heartland is filled with bigotry, homophobia, fear, and hatred somehow condoned by a religious interpretation. Certainly, though inaccurately, the church became the face of the heartland AIDS response in the eyes of those living on the coasts. However, I would argue that the counterprotesters Westboro inspired are much more reflective of the heartland AIDS response as a whole: a sometimes bizarre, almost always unlikely coalition of people who repurposed their unrelated skills (such as providing a loud motorcade to render the off-key songs of protesters inaudible, and crafting fabulous angel costumes that both honored the dead and protected their families from disrespect) to meet unexpected and unprecedented needs. If only in response to Phelps's intense homophobia and AIDS phobia, counterprotesters created home and belonging for those who been denied them and called on and refuted varied aspects of the white heartland imaginary.

Conclusion

The heartland response to the early AIDS crisis was infused with religion at every turn. Whether in rallying support or galvanizing bigotry, religious rhetoric and interpretation became the political language of AIDS in the region.[77] In an area synonymous with a sparse population, fierce independence, and religiosity, religious institutions and their outreach efforts provided most of the service organization and the political mobilizing apparatus for the entire region. From this perspective, the AIDS response had to become intertwined with religious activism, as religious organizations often owned the hospitals, coordinated social services, and had a consistent and unique communication opportunity every week in the form of a literal pulpit. By acknowledging and analyzing the role of religion in the heartland AIDS response, in the construction of positive and negative reactions to the epidemic, we also see how religious institutions and leaders not only used their religious interpretations but also deployed the white heartland imaginary to varying degrees and negotiated the right to home and belonging to support their religious justification for their reaction to the epidemic. While there is a relatively small but growing body of literature that explores religion in the AIDS crisis at the national level, the heartland example demands more grappling with how religion informed AIDS responses at the local, regional, and national levels.

CHAPTER FOUR
Medicine from the Ground Up

This chapter's analysis of the medical response to the HIV/AIDS epidemic in the heartland is a true culmination of the discussion in the previous chapters, in that we see an existing anemic medical infrastructure built on the white heartland imaginary, a reimagining of home and care among communities most impacted by the disease, and the centrality of religious institutions and rhetoric even in the scientific response. Though the facing image (figure 4.1) doesn't offer insight into the specific experiences of those fighting the AIDS crisis, it does illustrate the widespread and lasting effect of the white heartland imaginary on the medical infrastructure in the region. Several aspects of this photograph communicate the white heartland imaginary. First, the simple composition of the wide-open natural space with a fence and a handmade billboard communicates the natural ruggedness and wholesomeness associated with the white heartland imaginary while also emphasizing the importance of personal property (the fence) and hard work (the handmade billboard). Second, the content of the billboard itself is striking in all that it communicates with just four words—"I NEED A KIDNEY"—and a phone number. Certainly, the first suggestion here is desperation. However, of equal import for this chapter are the real and discursive backstories of the white heartland imaginary communicated by these four words: the failures of a larger public safety net in a pallid medical system, a poorly run organ donation system, and a startling self-sufficiency that takes neoliberal ideals to the extreme. Third is the use of the word "I"—"I need a kidney," not "Jim needs a kidney" or "Susan needs a kidney." "I need a kidney" illuminates an intense bootstrap mentality idolized by the very forces that deployed the white heartland imaginary most effectively in the 1980s. Here, a person who is so significantly impacted by a failing organ that they need a new one has seemingly built their own billboard and appears to be determined to manage their own medical care despite their illness. This extreme independence evoked by "I" is both the ideal and the failing of the white heartland imaginary and neoliberalism at large.

With the arrival of the AIDS crisis in the heartland, this disparate landscape becomes the backdrop for people so ill they are not able to build their own proverbial billboards, people for whom demanding greater support and medical care is the only feasible response, and the regional response deems

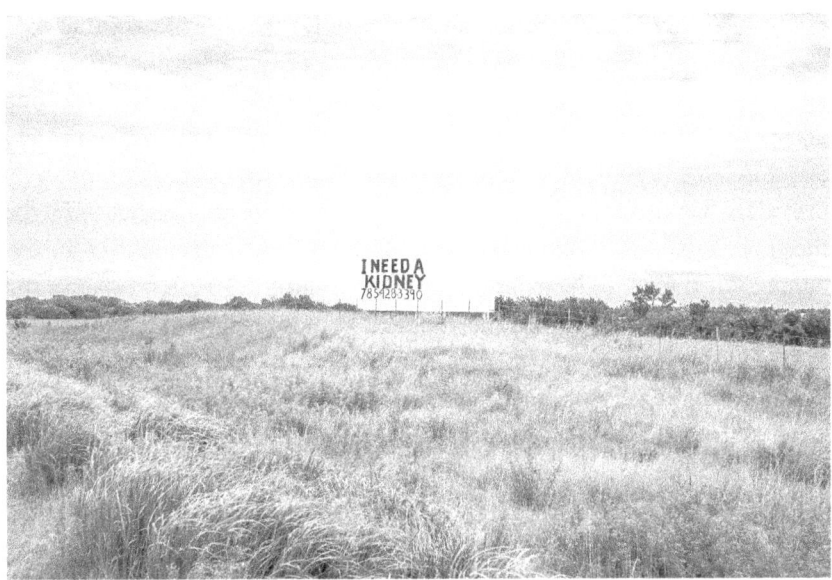

FIGURE 4.1 Philip Heying, *Repurposed Billboard West of Salina, Kansas, along I-70 7/13/2014—1:40 P.M*, 2014. Inkjet print. Spencer Museum of Art, University of Kansas, Museum purchase: Elmer F. Pierson Fund, 2018.0180.

illness a deserved punishment or an unspeakable moral failure, not an opportunity for compassion or increased resources. This chapter first traces the shadow of the white heartland imaginary on the regional medical response by looking at Dr. Donna Sweet of Wichita, Kansas, a literal one-woman regional AIDS response, who skillfully deploys her insider status as a part of the white heartland imaginary to expand healthcare for people with AIDS in the region. Then, medical outreach created by those denied access to the white heartland imaginary illustrates the renegotiation and reimagining of home among queer Black communities. Lastly, this chapter will turn to the role of individual medical institutions in meeting the real medical needs of those with HIV/AIDS in the region, building on the discursive landscape mapped out in chapter 3. Taken together, the medical response to HIV/AIDS in the heartland emerges as deeply informed by the white heartland imaginary and in the reimagining of home that is regionally specific in its extremism but also echoes to a lesser extent throughout the US AIDS response.

"Donna Sweet, the HIV Goddess of Kansas"

Though the AIDS epidemic presented itself slightly later and on a much smaller scale in the heartland region than in coastal cities, it also faced a vastly different medical terrain that significantly impacted the way that doctors and public health officials responded to the disease locally.[1] In this region where AIDS specialists were (and remain) rarities, often with just one doctor or just one social worker single-handedly representing the entirety of a state's medical AIDS response team, these providers emerge as not only providers but also activists, and not just for their city or state but often for the entire region. Dr. Donna Sweet of Wichita, Kansas, exemplifies the dynamism of the white heartland imaginary amid the HIV response in the heartland, the precarity of the medical response, and the blurring of the medical and activist divide against the landscape of the country's center.

Historians or activists would find it difficult to place a single person at the heart of the New York City or San Francisco AIDS response, without whom there would not have been a response. After all, no single person has provided healthcare to every single AIDS patient since the arrival of the epidemic in those cities; how could they? No single person spearheaded the city or state's AIDS-related housing crisis. No single person engaged the prison population in the HIV/AIDS response or traveled the state to give hundreds of educational presentations to everyone from elementary school children to infectious disease specialists and from rotary clubs to cosmetologist conventions. No single person coordinated nursing home care and annual fundraisers for expensive medications and held regular office hours in makeshift clinics spread out across hundreds of miles of sparsely populated terrain, requiring the coordination of crop dusters, private jets, church vans, and huge duffle bags filled with medical records and supplies. No single person in New York and San Francisco saw how AIDS-related legislation unintentionally excluded access to funding needed to care for their patients, learned how to lobby, and not only got the laws changed but continued to advise lawmakers and lobbyists at the local, state, and national levels more than thirty years later. In Kansas, one person did. Not one person for each of these issues; one person did them *all* at once, and still does, in stilettoes. She remains the only doctor in the state certified by the American Academy of HIV Medicine Specialists, and at various moments in the last forty years, she has also cared for patients in Colorado, Nebraska, North and South Dakota, and Montana as the closest certified provider.

Sweet's positionality to the white heartland imaginary and her personality proved to be as important as her medical training in addressing the state's epidemic in the state. She is truly tireless, indomitable, and a deft medical provider and thus, out of necessity, a political operator. Though this is a rare constellation of attributes to appear in the world, they seem to be fairly common characteristics, and perhaps even requirements, of doctors in the early AIDS crisis. However, Sweet stands in a much smaller subset of early AIDS care providers in her relationship to and awareness of the white heartland imaginary. She was as much of an "insider" as possible for a woman: "I'm born and bred not only Kansas but Wichita. I grew up on a farm about forty miles east [of Wichita] and was born in this hospital," where she now teaches and practices.[2] One of many children in a large, politically conservative family, she stayed close to home for her undergraduate and medical degrees before completing her postgraduate training in infectious diseases at the University of Kansas Wichita in 1982. She is fluent in Protestant and Catholic religious cultures and a familiar face amid the nonprofit community in the city and state, and she is only ever seen without high heels (though never without makeup) at an annual backyard fundraising picnic. In short, Donna Sweet embodied the white heartland imaginary that President Reagan deployed in the early 1980s to bolster his conservative revolution, Christian political morality, and neoliberal ideals of small state / big individual responsibility. Though more educated than the imagined ideal, she ticked nearly every other box: she was white, straight, gender conforming, and hard-working, had politically conservative roots, and was at least adjacent to farming, as well as financially successful, religious, and closely tied to her nuclear family, and she supported non-state-based service organizations. These characteristics, and the resulting legibility they garnered across the region, marking her as belonging and innocuous, gave her the ability to disarm those with AIDS phobia and effectively advocate and coordinate among those who existed easily in the white heartland imaginary.

AIDS first appeared on Sweet's radar when the hospital's infectious disease nurses invited her to give a talk, as a member of the University of Kansas medical school faculty, about the new disease in 1982, because of her interest in immunology. Though not an infectious disease specialist, she gathered all the research she could find on AIDS at the time, which was very little, and gave a talk, only to be asked to give it again numerous times. Quickly, she became established as "the AIDS doctor."[3] Her first patient with AIDS was a man who was moving home to be with his family after his diagnosis, and when word spread that he was looking for a doctor, Sweet thought, "I could do it as well as anybody else."[4] He was the first of hundreds. She explained that "early on, they were almost all come-homers," as opposed to homegrown cases, which increased over time.[5] A few months later, a man wandered into her clinic at the university medical center after arriving in Kansas from New York earlier that day to "visit" his family, who took him immediately to the hospital from the airport. He died within twenty-four hours, having never made it to his family's home, with Dr. Sweet having to inform the family that he had HIV. He was the first person to die from AIDS in the state of Kansas, and Dr. Sweet has treated every single person with HIV/AIDS in the state since then, over 1,300 patients.[6] Sweet described her early patients: "The bulk of the people that came to me were oftentimes people who grew up around here, went to the coasts to have a freer lifestyle and do different things and acquired . . . AIDS but ended up destitute and needing help so they would come back to the homeland . . . and everybody died in six to twelve months."[7] Though there were no treatments available for several years after those first cases, Dr. Sweet gained a reputation in the medical community and the communities most impacted by the disease as a thorough doctor who fought for her patients' care and comfort, as efficient but warm, a giver of big hugs and holder of hands for her patients, and a genteel arm-twister who would not take "no" from everyone else. She embraced this new role as the AIDS doctor in Kansas and pursued additional certification from the American Academy of HIV Medicine Specialists. From those early days of compiling and sharing research, Sweet's name was and is ubiquitous in HIV treatment in Kansas.

As she truly became an expert on HIV/AIDS and not just the only person who had seen a patient with AIDS, improving access to quality care became the highest priority for Sweet. As a first step, she instigated training for medical professionals around the state in HIV testing (once it was available in 1985) and care for stabilized patients. She joined the faculty at the University of Kansas Medical Center in Wichita and required all internal medicine residents to complete an HIV/AIDS rotation with her.[8] While there are many more doctors around the state who are competent at diagnosing and managing HIV/AIDS as a result of her ongoing efforts, especially now, with all the effective medications and prophylaxis, she remains to this day the only AIDS specialist in the state and currently has a caseload of well over 2,000, including every HIV-positive Kansan. Fortunately, as medicines have become more effective, she sees many of these patients only sporadically. Pharmacological advancements are not the only significant change to affect her ability to provide quality care. Rural healthcare has been transformed by the internet, electronic medical files, video chatting, and computer-based technologies over the last twenty years. However, in the years before these breakthroughs, Dr. Sweet's medical practice looked far different from those of her coastal and urban counterparts.

Starting in the late 1980s (and in some locations, continuing even today), Dr. Sweet worked with medical providers in a handful of Kansas locations to ensure that she had regular office hours to meet with HIV-infected patients who were not able to come to her clinic in Wichita. While this may not seem like a significant burden at first glance, the creation of these extension offices was a feat of political deftness and logistical skill. At one time and for several years, Dr. Sweet had five offices spread across the state in Pittsburg, Salina, Atchison, Wichita, and Garden City.[9] The simple logistics of running one of these clinics, let alone five, reveals the staggering amount of work Sweet and her career-long administrative assistant Sheryl Kelly did before seeing a single patient. Sweet explained, "Garden City was the difficult one. They had quite a few patients, a little bit different demographics: not gay, primarily Mexican, Central American, largely undocumented, and consequently were tough to get into care. . . . I just knew I couldn't drive there and back and give up as much time as it would take to do that."[10] In the late 1980s, Garden City was experiencing significant growth as immigrants from Asia and Latin America arrived in the town to work in the recently opened meatpacking plant, bringing the town's population to over 20,000 for the first time in its history. Roughly 200 miles from the three sizeable cities of Amarillo, Wichita, and Denver, Garden City is one of the largest towns in western Kansas and is now also one of the most racially diverse. It is home to one of the region's largest hospitals and has a regional airport just eight miles outside of town. This made it an obvious choice for an outpost for Sweet's outreach clinics.

As with many parts of the AIDS response in this region, the church proved pivotal in connecting people with HIV with services. Dr. Sweet learned about the existence of the United Methodist Mexican American Ministries clinic adjacent to St. Catherine's Hospital through conversations with colleagues at the University of Kansas, and she worked with them to set up a regular time when she could use their office space for appointments. Drawing on her religious background and making the most of her legibility as part of the white heartland imaginary, she worked with Methodist contacts in Wichita to initiate a relationship with the United Methodist Church in Garden City, not only to access office space for free but also to arrange for a church van to pick her and her team up at the airport and transport them to the clinic. She used these regular visits to see patients and also to educate general practitioners and the public in and around Garden City. With logistics largely in place on the ground in Garden City, that left only the question of how to get there. She recalled, "That's when I got the hare-brained idea to ask KU [the

University of Kansas] to use their plane, and they [agreed]. It was an in-kind donation to my grant."[11]

In the first fifteen years of the AIDS epidemic in Kansas, the medical response was held together by metaphorical duct tape, shoestrings, and goodwill, epitomized by the travel logistics undertaken by Sweet and her longtime administrative assistant Sheryl Kelly. At various points in the epidemic, depending on need, funding, and technology, she made regular trips to Garden City (as well as the other four clinic sites) at intervals ranging from every three weeks to every eight weeks. Funding for an AIDS response was extremely limited in the years before the Ryan White CARE Act of 1990, and even when it passed, Sweet had to stretch the few dollars she got across more patients and a much larger landscape than the legislation was designed to cover. On the multiple days of the week that she saw patients, she rose before the sun, put on makeup and high heels, and grabbed her three or four large black duffle bags eventually held together by duct tape at the seams. These duffle bags were her portable office, stuffed with patient charts, intake forms, educational pamphlets for providers, patients, and community members, any medical equipment she might need, all medications, and meals and snacks for herself and the variable team assembled for each trip, which could include her assistant, a nurse, a medical student, and/or a resident. She carpooled to the Wichita airport, where she often watched the sun rise while boarding either the KU plane or whatever plane she could wrangle to take her to one of her four outposts.[12] These planes were sometimes chartered planes paid for by other clinics or by grants for rural medicine initiatives in the state, which happened to be going to the same location and had a few untaken seats. It wasn't unusual for a member of her team to learn at the last minute that there wasn't enough room, and they would drive up to 200 miles to the clinic to meet Sweet there. When she could not arrange for one of these cushier options, she would work her connections in rural communities to arrange for a farmer to pick her up with his crop duster. However, there were also plenty of times when flight logistics didn't come together, and Sweet and her team would road-trip across the state, logging thousands of miles in 500- and 300-mile increments, driving to and from Garden City or Pittsburg or Salina, leaving Wichita before dawn, seeing patients for ten hours, staying in one of the few motels in town, and driving back to Wichita the next day, only to drive to another town later that week.[13] Even when she arrived in one of her outpost clinics, her journey could grow more complicated when patients too sick to journey to the outposts would need home visits, often requiring another impromptu crop duster flight, which provided both transportation and an inconspicuous arrival in a farming community where a person's HIV-positive status could draw significant stigma and raise safety concerns. Looking back, she shrugged and sighed, "They weren't going to get care otherwise."[14]

In addition to making regularly scheduled visits to clinics across the state, Sweet was also trying to find care for her patients when they left her clinic. This took tremendous advocacy, care, and education that was highly personalized to each patient. Perfectly illustrating this point, Sweet recalled:

> I had sent one of my patients back home to, I think, Ashland, Kansas. It was way west in western Kansas to a nursing home they had, and there was almost an uprising among the employees about accepting this patient. They were just petrified. To their credit, they were just scared to death. So, we made arrangements with one of their local rancher farmers that had a little plane. He came to Wichita, picked me up, and flew me back, and they had what they called euphemistically a grass landing strip, which is just you land in the pasture—one of my more hair-raising adventures. And I talked in the church there, I talked at the nursing home, and I talked in the school system. I think it made a difference. I made [sure] to touch the guy. I've always been a hugger and still am, but then it was important because these guys didn't get touched.[15]

Sweet's need-driven and innovative medical infrastructure relied on her deft redeployment and insurgent use of the white heartland imaginary. She knowingly used her insider status and the general acceptance of her "belonging" in the heartland to expand not only healthcare but the very definition of who could survive and sustain in the heartland as a site of home and living. Her history illuminates numerous aspects of the idiosyncrasies of the response to AIDS in the heartland that resonate far beyond Kansas, including the crucial role of doctors as activists, the importance of religious-based services, creative education efforts in politically conservative settings, and the practical deployments of limited resources, including farming tools like crop dusters. In terms of the larger history of AIDS and the heartland, Sweet shines a spotlight on the ways that white heartland ideals could be manipulated to work against their designed and deployed intention. She also oddly epitomizes certain aspects of the white heartland imaginary, apart from her race and marital status and other demographic information: she built an entire regional medical response to a pandemic and held it together, at times, with literal duct tape. On the one hand, she could be the poster woman for self-sufficiency and bootstrapping grit; on the other hand, the important reality is that she did it all for and with others, demonstrating an interdependency that flies in the face of neoliberal ideals.[16]

Reaching Out, Bringing In, and All Pulling Together

In 1990, Erise Williams was a regular on the dance floor at the Twist, one of three St. Louis gay bars that had either a Black night or a Black happy hour. He didn't care if he was dancing with anyone or not; he was always on the floor moving to the synthesized rhythms of the house music that was quickly gaining popularity among clubgoers across the country—"I was a club head," he says. It was at one of these Black nights at the Twist that another Black queer man approached Williams with a proposition. Virgil Grandberry worked in the St. Louis Public Health Department at the time and had also just founded a nonprofit called Blacks Assisting Blacks against AIDS (BABAA). When he saw Erise dancing, and the ease with which he mingled with others at the bar, Virgil realized that Erise was the man he had been looking for to get the word out about AIDS to the Black gay community. Grandberry pulled Williams aside and offered him a part-time job handing out educational pamphlets and condoms wherever he thought best. Williams recalled, "He [Grandberry] said that's why I want you, because people know you, and you go out a lot, and people are used to you." Erise agreed. He went to an American Red Cross training on HIV/AIDS and African Americans and met other activists, all women, working on AIDS in the Black community, who taught him how to initiate conversations about HIV. Williams then took these conversations to the clubs and Black queer men: "Especially in our community, there wasn't anyone else talking about it. . . . I even started talking to people on the bus and passing out condoms on the bus." At the time, many men of color assumed HIV/AIDS was a white man's disease, and disease prevention efforts often stopped at the advice to "not hav[e] sex with white men and not hav[e] sex with Black men who had sex with white men."[17] Grandberry wanted Williams and BABAA to be a more accurate, pervasive, and accessible source of education, outreach, and services specifically for Black men in St. Louis, southwestern Illinois, and eastern Missouri. When Grandberry himself succumbed to AIDS a little over a year later, in 1992, Williams stepped in as the new executive director of BABAA and got additional funding from the St. Louis AIDS Foundation, and slowly BABAA became one of the largest AIDS service organizations specifically for men of color in the heartland. For the next decade, until 2002, Williams built a creative network of outreach programs, services, and a strong community of people of color to respond to the AIDS crisis.

Before delving into the innovative healthcare and home-making strategies BABAA came to embody to engage queer men of color in the AIDS discussion, it is critical to first put Williams, Black queer St. Louisans, and BABAA into the context of the heartland white imaginary and understandings of home. Like most cities in the United States, St. Louis is intensely racially segregated, with Delmar Boulevard acting as the city's dividing line. Though the city has a very rich Black history and queer history, these histories remain just beneath the surface for many, especially those who never or rarely cross Delmar Boulevard and live in the overwhelmingly white sections of the city. Thus, St. Louis offers insight into how the white heartland imaginary works to erase the very existence of people of color by simply zooming out far enough or centering its gaze on white spaces. However, for people of color, and especially queer folks of color, the landscape molded by the white heartland imaginary required a careful choreography of movement and creative means of developing and maintaining community. For example, Williams's presence on that dance floor in the nightclub wasn't random. Williams reminisced, "Knights and Magnolia's both had a Black night. Knights had a Saturday happy hour from like 5 to 9, and . . . the segregation in the city was even down to that level where at 5 o'clock, the club became Black: they played house music, and it was mostly Black people. And at 9 o'clock, you could see the Black guys leaving and white guys coming in. Very segregated. The music changed, all of that at the same time."[18] Whiteness permeated the city, even in spaces designated as Black. Black bar patrons knew when their time was up and they needed to vacate spaces. This level of segregation, although it was not codified into law, is reminiscent of the Jim Crow South or sundown towns. Yet, these fleeting moments and spaces were critical to the Black queer men pushed to the peripheries of both the Black and queer communities. In short, Black queer men were denied entry to the white heartland imaginary on multiple fronts, which often translated into temporary and tenuous access to spaces to call home or community sites.

The addition of the AIDS epidemic to these already precarious and carefully negotiated claims to spaces and services added further complexity. To be clear, the earliest, predominantly white organizations formed in response to HIV/AIDS were technically welcoming to everyone, but they did no specific outreach or services to engage men of color directly, embracing a color-blind approach to service provision. Even as the local epidemic began to impact women of color more disproportionately, some organizations, like DOORWAYS, sought to reach out and intentionally design services for women of color, deploying respectability based on heterosexuality to make their efforts more palatable to the larger community. Similarly, Black-facing community organizations like A Better Family Life emphasized heterosexuals—"They never ever really touched Black LGBT folks," and "were very slow to get onboard" with HIV/AIDS.[19] Cathy Cohen, Darius Bost, and Dan Royles have written extensively about the respectability politics at work in Black communities in the 1980s and 1990s that often resulted in minimizing or completely overlooking LGBTQ Black existence.[20] There were important organizations like BABAA that stand in stark contrast to this, but the force of respectability politics as a direct offshoot of the white heartland imaginary blunted the St. Louis AIDS response for Black queer community members. Thus, queer people of color never garnered the devoted attention of the larger organizations in the city as they were denied claims to the white heartland imaginary based on their race and their sexuality.

Making matters worse, as queer men of color became a quickly increasing demographic of infection, the existing (white) organizations and career activists declared themselves capable of meeting their needs without changing their services, often denying queer men of color positions on staffs and boards of directors. However, those services failed to engage the Black queer community in any meaningful way that would communicate their increased risk or their belonging in the AIDS response spaces. White organizations and service providers failed at being culturally competent among people of color: "They don't understand why it's important that somebody who looks like them and who understands their culture is important. . . . They saw themselves at odds [with BABAA] because they had created agencies and careers, and it's about keeping and maintaining those. . . . They [white organizations] have been culturally conditioned to think if something is all Black, then somehow it's not for me."[21] Consequently, the St. Louis AIDS response initially became another extension of the white heartland imaginary, actively denying members of minoritized communities access to a sense of belonging or home, even within spaces that included them and with regard to issues that impacted them deeply.

Grandberry designed BABAA with the specific intention of meeting Black queer folks where they were physically and socially, using Black culture to create a sense of belonging, and ultimately building new sites of home, family, and community that defied the white heartland imaginary. Grandberry had initially scraped together money from public health funds and minor local grants to hire Williams as a part-time community outreach health worker. Under the Clinton administration, changes to the federal funding of HIV/AIDS organizations that earmarked certain funds for organizations with predominantly racial minority boards, staff, and clientele allowed BABAA to grow quickly under Williams's tenure as executive director.[22] Williams, along with an innovative staff and board of directors, implemented long-lasting and meaningful health interventions that simultaneously deepened Black queer ties to the heartland as a site of home. What started with Williams personally handing out condoms on the St. Louis buses and at Black dance nights and happy hours at the Twist, Knights, and Magnolia's eventually culminated in St. Louis hosting what is now the second-oldest Black Pride celebration in the United States, among other significant programs.

Williams and BABAA harnessed Black cultural phenomena to connect AIDS resources and testing with Black queer people. James Earl Hardy's book *B-Boy Blues*, published in 1994, epitomized the vibrant cultural movement that grappled with the intersections of Blackness and AIDS in numerous artistic forms ranging from fiction and film to music and dance.[23] Williams explained, "The culture was just booming, and it was because of this epidemic and because we as Black gay men found our voice. . . . We found a space for us. We knew we could no longer be silent."[24] Williams saw the emerging Black gay culture and the necessary response to AIDS within the community as deeply intertwined. The connection to these cultural markers allowed BABAA to grow its outreach in unexpected ways for an AIDS organization. "If there was any benefit from the AIDS epidemic, it was Black and Latino men starting to define themselves as themselves, not so much assimilating to their white counterparts in the white LGBTQ community, but defining and shaping their communities, developing a style, even the way they dressed and danced."[25]

The first B-Boy Festival was steeped in several cultural art forms, as it consisted of a book signing by Hardy followed by a festival emceed by local drag celebrity Vicky Valentino in a specific area popular among the city's Black and Latino men in Forest Park, one of the largest parks in the city: picnic areas 11 and 12. Williams remembers, "Even at our first B-Boy Festival, we had a vogueing contest" and a ball competition, as organizers recognized that the established ballroom and vogueing culture among Black queer men in St. Louis and across the country offered a way to gain access to this specific population of low-income, queer men of color.[26] "In our efforts to continue to work with that population and get to know that population, we started supporting them by having a B-Boy Festival and having a vogue contest as part of our outreach. We would do the festival, and we would have a table there to talk about HIV/AIDS, and we were offering testing, and people were getting tested. And the attendance was anywhere from 300 to 600 people, and we would be in Forest Park until they put us out."[27] By embracing and creating these cultural art forms and celebrations, BABAA became incredibly adept at creating cultural events at which queer men of color felt safe and had a sense of belonging, and then integrating AIDS education and testing into those events. At one point, BABAA ran a hip-hop dance troop (the B-Boys of BABAA) that would go into high schools to dance and provide AIDS education in a mock Jerry Springer forum to engage the youth—a program that ultimately was invited to perform at the National HIV Prevention Conference in Washington, DC. The B-Boy Festival served as the precursor to the city's Black Pride Festival, which continues today. In a city where spaces specifically for queer of color bodies were often impermanent exceptions, BABAA created several annual events that temporarily transformed public spaces into queer men of color spaces that were highly anticipated and strongly attended. For a community intentionally and repeatedly denied validation, acknowledgment, and a sense of belonging, BABAA became a careful crafter of home that reflected the vibrant Black queer culture that permeated the 1990s. This work offered a site of refuge and moments of reprieve but also undermined the larger political work of the white heartland imaginary by centering community, Blackness, and queerness.

While events like the B-Boy Festival were important first steps in creating a sense of belonging and home for Black queer men in St. Louis, Williams wanted a permanent community center that would negate the need to borrow private spaces or coordinate the use of public spaces for events. With funding from both federal and local grants, BABAA opened its community center, which it called Harambee. *Harambee* is a Swahili word meaning "all pulling together"; it is a guiding principle in Kenya (the word appears on the national flag) that evokes a community pulling together to help itself, a sort of communal self-help model. Whereas the neoliberal notion of bootstrapping individualism anchored the white heartland imaginary, Harambee was a very intentional unraveling and challenging of those concepts. BABAA's Harambee, which opened in 2000, was "one of the area's first drop-in centers for MSM, men who have sex with men."[28] While these services certainly met the specific needs of those who entered the center, Harambee offered the larger Black queer community something far more difficult to find amid the white heartland imaginary: home. Even DOORWAYS, the St. Louis AIDS housing organization discussed in chapter 3, had reinforced various aspects of the white heartland imaginary as they offered spaces to people with AIDS, first by assuming all clients would be young white gay men and then by deploying a different sort of respectability politics as it turned its attention to mothers and other women of color. Harambee was one of the few places unequivocally and unapologetically for Black queer men, offering an important reimaging of home in a heartland white imaginary that generally denied Black men of color any sense of belonging. At Harambee, Black men who had sex with men, whether they defined themselves as gay or not, "could come together, get a meal. We developed an advisory board, which some of the young men became a part of, to brainstorm new outreach methods. We had dances and BBQs. We were just building community. . . . It meant a lot to the young men."[29] On a small scale, it was undermining the white heartland imaginary, crafting home where there was not one and a diverse community where homogeneity reigned.

While Harambee and BABBA were integral to creating claims to home for Black queer men, even the homes and spaces designed to defy the white heartland imaginary had limits. In 2002, BABAA closed its doors as its creative outreach efforts, funding woes, and the racism and homophobia that saturated the white heartland imaginary came together in an explosive mix. Between 1990 and 2002, BABAA had grown to employ a staff of over forty, and it had an outreach office in East St. Louis and programs ranging from providing HIV testing and distributing condoms at bars to organizing the Black Pride events and running Harambee. However, federal programs became more flexible about their funding going to "minority-serving" agencies rather than "predominantly minority" agencies under the second Bush administration, meaning that more predominantly white organizations competed for the same funds. Consequently, some of BABAA's largest grants of the previous decade were set to expire in early 2002 without funds in place to make up the shortfall.[30] This was a direct result of the intensive abstinence-only funding limitations agencies like the CDC had to adhere to under the George W. Bush presidency. As a result, Williams made the difficult decision to lay off a handful of staff, including one person whose vengeance would ultimately bring about the end of BABAA by the end of the year.

Even with fewer staff to coordinate, July 2002 saw another BABAA innovative outreach effort: a safe-sex house party hosted by a well-known Black porn star, Sir Bobby Blake, who was also a safe-sex trainer at the Red Cross in Memphis, Tennessee.[31] Sir Bobby Blake was a frequent celebrity at similar events across the country. At these parties, which were common on the coasts, public health workers would collaborate with community groups or

Medicine from the Ground Up 91

celebrities to talk about safe-sex practices in a fun, direct, and social way, with a party to follow. Far less common in St. Louis than in cities like San Francisco or New York, safe-sex parties in St. Louis were typically conservative by comparison, despite their evocative name. BABAA used some of the funds from a CDC safe-sex education grant to pay the safe-sex instructor (in this case, Sir Bobby Blake), as was typical in almost all of its outreach efforts. However, the disgruntled former employee falsely claimed to local and national news outlets that Blake had stripped at the event and demonstrated different sexual acts as part of the educational component of the evening.[32] The consequences were swift and fierce: Erise Williams was forced to resign despite his objections, BABAA lost all of its CDC funding, and BABAA folded—all in a matter of weeks.

While BABAA is certainly far from the first community organization to close because of mismanagement or alleged mismanagement of federal grants, I think it is important to consider BABAA's experience in light of the white heartland imaginary at the local and national levels. Up until the Sir Bobby Blake safe-sex party, BABAA had garnered national attention and accolades for its innovative use of Black culture and Black cultural icons to craft a sense of belonging and a variety of services and outreach programs, all while building the largest Black AIDS service agency in the heartland. In serving the Black queer community, Williams had to thread a fine needle between drawing in Black queer clients who other interventions failed to reach and avoiding the wrath of the increasingly restrictive white heartland imaginary, especially as it began to conflate white heartland ideals with the abstinence-only ideals of the Bush administration.

Much of BABAA's success hinged on its and Williams's low profile but positive reputation in St. Louis and its ability to craft a sense of positive belonging for those left out of the white heartland imaginary without drawing too much attention, by focusing on prevention, testing, and services, and not on the failures of the white heartland imaginary and the existing organizations' inability to meet the needs of queer men of color. However, the very public story about a Black AIDS organization, a Black gay porn star, a "safe-sex house party," and a disgruntled former employee paved a short and easy path to a catastrophic scandal for BABAA. Although Williams and many others in attendance at the party contested the description of the night's events, BABAA could not pull itself back from the line it had purportedly crossed. In Williams's telling, "Long story short, that really hurt because besides it not being true, it really questioned my reputation to other people."[33] The white heartland imaginary demanded respectability, especially from those whose very existence was inconsistent with its basic premise.

Williams's next, post-BABAA career iteration reflected an understanding of these unspoken rules of the white heartland imaginary. In plotting his next move, which would ultimately lead to opening a health center for minorities in the city, Williams and Associates, "we knew that we couldn't continue to address HIV in a vacuum. We needed to reach out to other health issues and other health disparities. . . . How do we talk about HIV in a way that is more palatable to the people we are trying to reach? So we came up with the idea of let's just talk about health because there are health disparities especially Black people face every day," which could open a dialogue to also talk about sexual health. With this tack away from addressing AIDS directly among queer Black men, "we found that it did make it more palatable for folks. People were willing to talk about it rather than us just standing under a banner of just AIDS, because of the stigma.[34]" Not only did the larger community of people of color feel more welcome at Williams and Associates than at the gay-affiliated BABAA, but this tactic also clashed less with larger white heartland imaginary ideals like respectability and heterosexuality. Still, Williams used the cover of the more wide-reaching health organization to maintain much of BABAA's work. BABAA continues as a program folded into Williams and Associates, and though the Harambee drop-in center no longer exists, another drop-in community center has taken its place, the Rustin Center, named after gay civil rights leader Bayard Rustin and created specifically for men experiencing housing precarity. In these ways, the sense of belonging and sites of home that BABAA created persist, but in more protected ways,

Medical Institutions and "Naughty Nuns"

The hospital infrastructure of the heartland in the 1980s reflected the warring ideals of conservative political ethos and social construction of the white heartland imaginary on one side and the dedication to science and religion on the other.[35] Hospitals were on the front lines of the shrinking social safety net at the heart of neoliberalism as they saw access and funding for medical care decrease as need simultaneously increased due to the erasure of other social programs and the onset of the HIV/AIDS epidemic. This was true across the country, but the very few private hospitals and the meager offerings of most public rural hospitals in the heartland landscape put the experiences of two specific types of hospitals into greater focus: those affiliated with university medical schools and those with religious affiliations. These hospitals played the greatest roles in addressing AIDS in the heartland, but in very different ways. While hospitals associated with medical schools approached HIV/AIDS as an area for research as well as a potential site for innovative care development, religiously affiliated hospitals, particularly those with ties to the Catholic Church and run by nuns, brought a religiously inspired compassion to patients with HIV/AIDS.

As the National Institutes of Health (NIH), Centers for Disease Control (CDC), and the Food and Drug Administration (FDA) became invested in developing a vaccine for HIV/AIDS in the early 1990s, a handful of medical schools and minority-specific community health centers across the country became important sites for vaccine trials. In the heartland, where the number of large university-affiliated hospitals is significantly smaller than on the coasts due to the smaller population, those that did gain access to vaccine trials played a significant role in the regional landscape. Washington University (Wash U) and St. Louis University (SLU), both in St. Louis, proved to be regional beacons for AIDS vaccine trials, just as the University of Kansas's medical campus in Wichita became the unexpected epicenter for patient care. Meanwhile, the University of Nebraska became an important location for drug development and, later, gene editing.[36] While these hospitals each contributed in important ways to the larger history of HIV/AIDS in the United States and globally, I will leave much of those histories for historians of science to uncover and explore. Instead, I want to situate these hospitals, specifically those that ran vaccine trials, as critical sites in the crafting of home and a sense of belonging for those typically denied home in the white heartland imaginary.

In February 1991, Rodney Wilson sat in the basement of the St. Louis Metropolitan Community Church (MCC) listening to a presentation by a nurse from the nearby SLU medical campus. At the time, Wilson had lost friends to AIDS and had found community in the openly LGBTQ-affirming MCC, but he remained in the closet in his professional life as a high school history teacher. He was looking for ways to be involved in the AIDS response without putting his career at risk. He remembered learning about the vaccine trials from the nurse, who was looking for vaccine trial participants to volunteer: "When you're young like that, you really do want to make a difference . . . so I was looking to do something that would be bigger than I was, help in a way that I could never imagine helping otherwise, so I made an appointment and went up to the campus there on Grand, the SLU hospital. . . . Yeah, I did it."[37] He ultimately spent three years volunteering as a vaccine trial participant, going through two eighteen-month trials. Every four to six weeks, he would drive to the hospital, get the injection, give blood samples, and report any potential side effects. Though the trials were double-blind, meaning that neither the doctors nor the patients knew if they were receiving the vaccine at the time, Wilson learned at the end of the trials that he had been given a placebo vaccine in one trial and a real, though ineffective, vaccine in the other. An HIV/AIDS vaccine remains elusive as we near the fiftieth anniversary of HIV's emergence, but being a vaccine trial participant gave Wilson a meaningful yet private way to contribute to the AIDS effort, especially as it was a role that was purposefully anonymous by design of the medical study so that participating did not out him like other forms of activism might have.

Fueled by its value and its safety (both in terms of disease transmission and remaining in the closet), Wilson became involved in SLU's community action board (CAB). Each vaccine site had a CAB because of the demands and protests of ACT UP activists on the coasts. Each CAB was to reflect the diversity of the community and advocate on its behalf, so "any new protocol that they were developing, we would read over for clarity of content, ease of read, or full disclosure of what was happening in a way that was easy to understand. We were looking out for the community, the volunteers, that was our job. We were there to be an eye on the process, the procedures, the protocols, to be certain that everyone who participated in these studies was fully informed and well educated about what the study was designed to do and how the study would work."[38] In both of these capacities, as a vaccine trial participant and CAB member, Wilson found a community of support and a way of giving back for a gay man not able to come out. Within a few months of beginning to work with these groups, Wilson officially came out at the high school where he taught and then fought for the celebration of LGBTQ History Month, which was front-page news in several local newspapers. As he fought to maintain his job and make changes to the curriculum, his standing in the community became a focus of public interest. Here, we see not that Wilson's work in the vaccine trials was important not only because it contributed to the fight against AIDS but also because it bestowed on him a sort of respectability through his association with the prominent local medical school and the selfless act of vaccine trial development. Although it was far from a motivating force for Wilson, the resulting respectability—along with his race, gender, religious affiliation, and class—allowed him some reprieve from the ostracizing power of the white heartland imaginary.

The presentation in the basement of the MCC of St. Louis that precipitated Wilson's involvement in the vaccine trials also exemplifies the many ways that religion factored into the medical response in somewhat unexpected ways, including in actual hospitals. More than any other religion in the region, Catholicism played a significant role in the AIDS response via Catholic-affiliated hospitals. I want to be clear here that there were only a handful of religions affiliated with hospitals in the region, and of those, the greatest number were Catholic hospitals that proved important to the care of people with AIDS. I am not trying to suggest that the Catholic Church had the best response to AIDS overall, a notion that has been impugned in many protests on both coasts and elsewhere. I also want to make an important distinction about the centrality of nuns in the Catholic AIDS response. Though some cardinals, like Cardinal May of St. Louis, were at times involved on a larger scale, nuns were often the sole representatives of the Catholic Church who saw AIDS activism and care as an extension of their faith. Priests of the heartland are conspicuously absent in the AIDS response, whether out of fear of being associated with homosexuality or simply because their duties did not grant them easy access to healthcare settings. In any case, nuns were often the crafters of care for people with AIDS in the heartland, in large part because nuns ran the Catholic hospitals.

As hospital administrators, nuns wielded significant power: they could make policies about caring for people with HIV/AIDS; they could coordinate with convents across the region to arrange for housing and care after discharge; they could provide free meeting space to local AIDS organizations; and they could mobilize the larger community to respond to those in need. In Topeka, Kansas, "almost all of the patients were at [the Catholic hospital] St. Francis, and the nuns were amazingly supportive. . . . They would take patients in, and if there wasn't a safe [place to] discharge [them], they would let them stay there for months, with no hope of getting paid anything more than a very small portion."[39] The same hospital was also home to the Topeka AIDS Project.

Even for those patients who either could not find a hospital to take them or had no means of caring for themselves at the end of life, religious groups, particularly Catholic nuns, played a major role. Wichita, Kansas, the same city where Donna Sweet was based, was also home to the Adorers of the Blood of Christ order of nuns, who were often on the very front lines of providing care during the final stages of life for AIDS patients. The order owned several buildings in the city, one of which they thought could be best used as a sort of hospice house for AIDS patients, run by an organization called

ConnectCare, for which the provincial of the order served as a member of the board of directors. One nun recalled, "This was the principal AIDS agency in Wichita at the time and had been founded by hospice [workers] because hospice was really not set up to take care of the really sick and dying young men."[40] Two sisters of the order, Sister Teresa Wetta and Sister Angela Houska, helped bring ConnectCare to fruition and "the AIDS House was one of our properties and we rented it to ConnectCare for a dollar a year or something like that."[41]

While Donna Sweet provided treatment and intervention, Erise Williams provided education and support services, and medical schools developed drugs and vaccines, a handful of nuns from the Adorers of the Blood of Christ were providing palliative care to a small handful of the many men who had no one else at the end of their battle with AIDS. The AIDS House, which was in operation from early 1993 to 2003, housed seven patients at a time, handpicked by Donna Sweet, who by then had been almost canonized and set on a pedestal: "She was just wonderful and she always moved very, very fast. We couldn't keep up with her."[42] Those in the AIDS House "were just the poorest and sickest. They were the ones who had no family support. In the early days, when you came there, it was pretty much to die, and you were grateful to have a warm place and food and to not have to worry about the bills anymore. . . . They [the patients] came and went pretty fast."[43]

Sister Joann Stuever joined the order in her retirement from her career as a science teacher after her children had finished college, her husband had passed, and her AIDS activism had already taken form, inspired by the AIDS Quilt and her HIV-positive brother. During the process of "discerning," or deciding whether to become a nun, which takes several years, Sister Joann assumed one of her first jobs for the order when she moved to Wichita in 1993:

> I found this dream job. I was the house mother at the AIDS House for seven very sick young men. I was the weekend house mother. I came Friday evening and went home Sunday afternoon. I lived with them, I cooked for them, I cleaned for them, washed dishes, planned menus, ordered groceries, organized volunteers to visit with them, play games, just give them some outside contact. Our beds were always full. It did involve hands-on care. I took people to the bathroom. . . . Dr. Sweet was their doctor, and she said, "They can eat anything they want. They need to be fattened up. Give them lots of butter-rich, cream-rich food. Cook up a storm and make a lot of desserts. We're

trying to keep the guys from losing weight so fast!" So that's what I did. . . . It was hard work. It was hard to be with them. . . . They were lonely. . . . They wanted to talk about relationships. They wanted to remember their families. I did a lot of listening. There was a lot of anger, a lot of hurt about being rejected, and one of my principal jobs was to sit and listen and hold hands.[44]

While all medical care is hard, especially in a lethal pandemic without any highly effective treatment or cure, palliative care for young men deeply stigmatized, ostracized, and dying long before they should have required a special kind of person, and often nuns answered the call.

While they did the challenging work of caring for these men, they were not just fighting HIV/AIDS; the nuns of the AIDS House in Wichita were also uniquely positioned to observe the machinations of the white heartland imaginary and the labor of building a final home in spite of it. The hard edges of the white heartland imaginary became backlit by the family tensions of the men in the AIDS House: "The few families I had interactions with were, 'We won't have anything to do with him. Don't put his last name in the paper when he dies.' The shame and the rejection was a large part of it."[45] The shame and resulting rejection were in large part a product of the white heartland imaginary, the homophobia it inspires, and the self-sufficiency and haleness it required, especially of men, but which men in the AIDS House could not perform because of their illness. Here we see the meeting of the discursive and the material effects of the white heartland imaginary playing out as a nun sits by the bedsides of dying men. Sister Joann remembered some of the hardest conversations:

> They wanted to talk about God. Almost to the man, they all felt that they were terrible sinners, that they deserved what they got, that AIDS was the punishment for their sins, and that they were going straight to hell when they died. And I would try to dissuade them of that notion and talk about that God is a loving God and it does not matter what they do, that God still loves them. And they could not wrap their heads around that. . . . There was not a day that went by that I did not tell them that they were beautiful and that I loved them and that God loved them. They just thought I was crazy.[46]

Much like these moments reveal the convergence of the discursive and material, they also reveal how the final stage of a deadly disease is not just a medical event but also deeply spiritual and often religious. In this region where religion played such an important role in both the imagined and real lives of those who lived here, Sister Joann's recollections are striking.

The experience was helpful to Sister Joann in finding distinctions between Catholic teachings and official responses to AIDS and her work at the AIDS House. In addition to running the house, ConnectCare also ran a food bank, organized monthly potlucks for the socialization of its clients, and coordinated the assembly and delivery of safe-sex kits (which included condoms and information about proper use and disposal) to Wichita bars. Sister Joann choked out a memory amid gales of laughter: "My greatest fear was that I would be driving around transporting a big cardboard box of these things and I would be sideswiped at an intersection or T-boned, and my car would flip over and out would come all these condoms, and it would be in the *Wichita Eagle* [the local newspaper]!" But in reality, her work was often in flagrant noncompliance with Catholic teachings against condom use due to the sanctity of life, especially since the initial statement on AIDS written in Archbishop May's time had long been replaced by the much more conservative "Called to Compassion and Responsibility."[47] She recalled grappling with the anti-condom stance: "Wait a minute. Let's think about our community. How many of them are getting pregnant anyhow? There were a lot of us who just saw the fallacy in the whole thing and just decided to do what our hearts told us to do. . . . This is not birth control. This is disease prevention."[48] Here we see in this personal navigation of religious rules and beliefs the nuances of religion on which the heartland AIDS response relied in very real ways and on scales both large and small.

Conclusion

This closer examination of the regional medical responses reveals the extent to which the white heartland imaginary saturated and influenced the lived experiences of those fighting against AIDS in the region. We see the white heartland imaginary as the specter that frightened families away from their dying sons, gave nuns nightmares of condom-strewn crash scenes, fueled deathbed existential crises, and shut down the largest Black AIDS service organization in the region, practically overnight. However, we also see the deployment of the white heartland imaginary's favorite currency, respectability, to bolster support, deliver care, and fill vaccine trials. Undoubtedly, the white heartland imaginary is overwhelmingly a tool of oppression, but the medical landscape of the heartland AIDS response also reveals inventive agency at work.

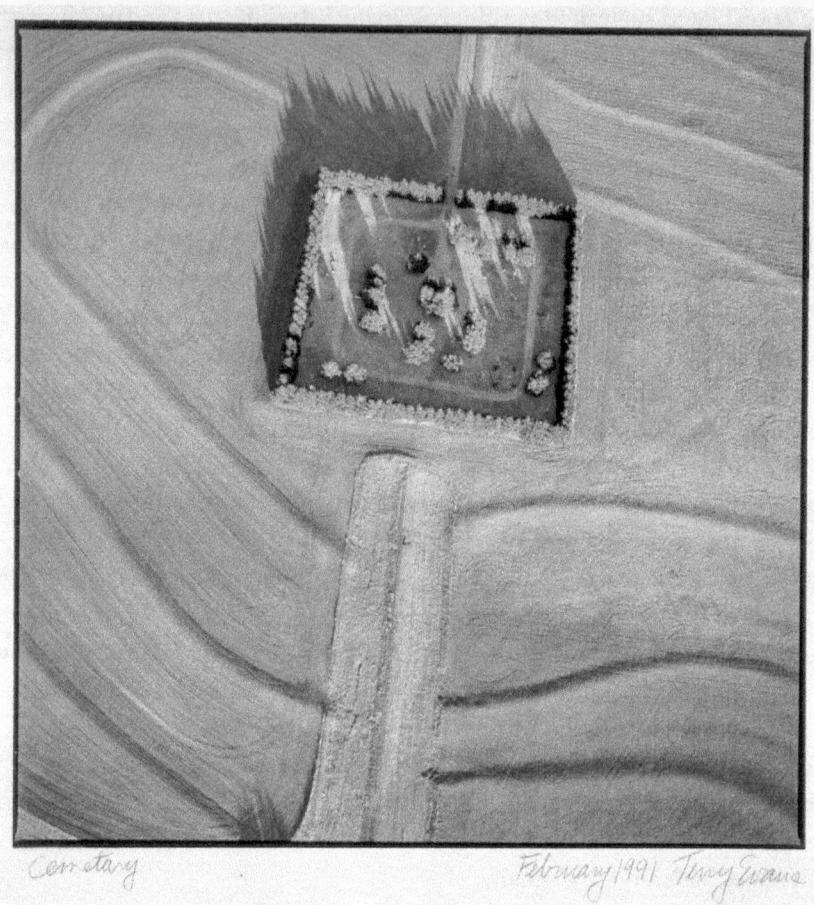

FIGURE 4.2 Terry Evans, *Cemetery, February 1991*. Gelatin silver print. Spencer Museum of Art, University of Kansas, Museum purchase: Helen Foresman Spencer Art Acquisition Fund, 1992.0032.

The failings, or lacunae, of the existing AIDS historiography also come into greater focus through the lens of the medical responses in the heartland. Like the photograph of a farm cemetery above (figure 4.2), the existing literature portrays the heartland AIDS experience as small, contained, tragic, easily overlooked, and almost always flown over. However, this picture also reveals a shadow seeping out across a terrain more nuanced than expected, and the cemetery itself looks well trodden, cared for, and more dynamic than this one angle can reveal. The same is true of the lessons offered by the heartland medical response. For one, few contemplate how a rural landscape might complicate any kind of healthcare, let alone the early AIDS crisis.

BABAA's work stands in contrast to the notion that the heartland is populated only by white people and that innovative activism could originate or appear only on the coasts. While much of our society sets up a binary of religion or science, this history demands a broader spectrum, greater nuance, so that ACT UP activists in New York can stage die-ins in St. Patrick's Cathedral and Sister Joann can regale visitors to the convent with tales of the old annual ART AID fundraisers they held to fund the AIDS House, at which "they would always put the nuns right down front at the end of the runway so they could throw roses at us and stuff like that. It was great fun. They loved us and they knew the whole AIDS House wouldn't be there without us. The nuns were revered, held in awe . . . and we educated a lot of nuns, HA!"[49]

CHAPTER FIVE
Political Posturing

Politics, as much as virology, drove the regional and national response to HIV/AIDS in the last two decades of the twentieth century. Ultimately, this book argues that the neoliberal and assimilationist responses to HIV/AIDS in the heartland resonated with the white heartland imaginary in such ways that they became the blueprint for LGBTQ politics in the late twentieth- and early twenty-first-century United States nationally. In short, the (re)deployment and contestation of the white heartland imaginary was the tactic that became more widely adopted and replicated by the larger LGBTQ movement than the refusal and total reimagining of the heartland or notions of home. The ways the white heartland imaginary was culturally produced and mobilized externally through the Reagan administration and popular culture, and internally via local activists leveraging proximity to white heartland imaginary ideals to gain palatability, validity, and support, reflect the kind of neoliberalism that Ruth Wilson Gilmore calls "organized abandonment."[1] The version of the HIV/AIDS response in the heartland that left the white heartland imaginary largely unchallenged inspired and fueled the dominant approach in LGBTQ politics nationally in the period between 1990 and 2015.

However, I cannot just corroborate this homonormative turn and monolithic understanding of queer politics as increasingly assimilationist and reliant on respectability in the waning decades of the twentieth century and the start of the twenty-first. The history of AIDS in the heartland also complicates and challenges this existing historiography. I want to be very clear: radical politics and activism existed and still exist in the heartland. The tactics that had worked at the local level to grant the more radical organizations power to shape the larger landscape shrank as the political scale shifted from local to national. Much like the train in the facing image (figure 5.1), the powerful motion takes on greater meaning up close and fades as the perspective widens to the full landscape. This chapter explores this political nuance and the tactical moves of radical organizations at the local level and illustrates the ongoing theft and reclamation of home in the heartland that lies at the heart of AIDS activism in the region.

For this chapter, I define politics as actions that try to expand or preserve the personal rights and safety of individuals and minoritized groups. Using

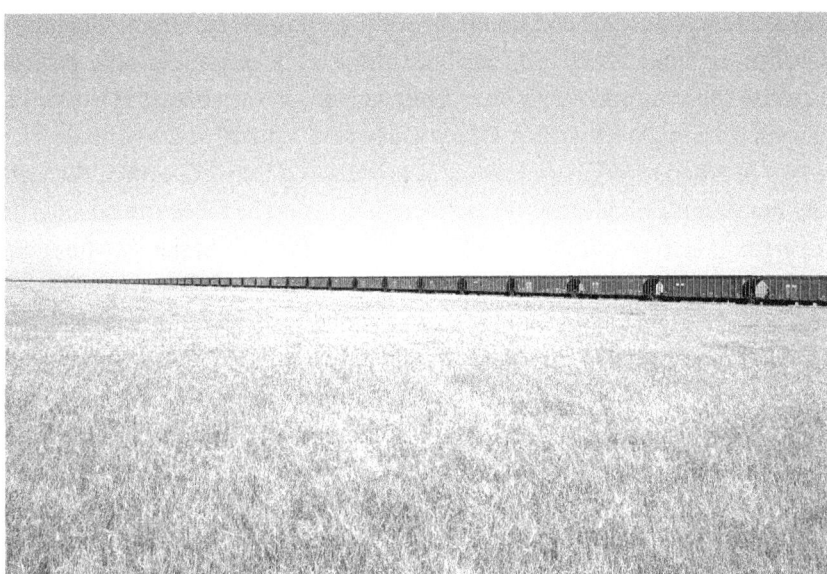

FIGURE 5.1 Larry Schwarm, *Empty Train Cars in Wheat Field near Friend, Kansas, May 2012*. Inkjet print. Courtesy of Larry Schwarm.

this definition, I explore political activism in two forms: first, activism fighting to protect or increase legal rights and protections for those with HIV/AIDS; and second, activism dismantling AIDS phobia and stigma through education. Even as a wide range of activist tactics and political framings emerge in these two realms, they are all in conversation with the white heartland imaginary. Some seek to claim inclusion or proximity to the white heartland imaginary without much expansion of it, some seek to use their proximity to white heartland ideals to expand the imaginary to garner support for AIDS activism, and others problematize the white heartland imaginary and offer a reimagining of home. However, even those who imagine new homes and new heartlands that are more inclusive of their needs and the needs of the AIDS epidemic are in conflict with the white heartland imaginary, the larger neoliberal pressures, and the history of the amorphous heartland landscape. Politics in the heartland barters for rights almost entirely within existing systems, whereas attaining justice through a reimagination of those systems is relegated to the peripheries, often deemed not possible from the outset.

Privacy emerges as the terrain of contestation for all these activists working within the white heartland imaginary. Privacy is a complex concept that is at once deeply imbricated with the state and the public (which define the

Political Posturing 103

parameters of privacy) and simultaneously supposedly free from state interference or public view. So, what we think of as private is only private because the state and public have deemed it so. In the context of the white heartland imaginary and AIDS, privacy is a salient political tool. The white heartland imaginary celebrates privacy as a freedom earned through the successful embodiment of neoliberalism using the following calculus: If a person is self-sustaining, which is made significantly easier by whiteness and other structural privileges, they deserve privacy; if they are reliant on the state or larger community, they are justifiably surveilled and denied privacy. Those deploying the white heartland imaginary for national political gain offered up the promise of privacy, often equated with freedom, as the prize for the successful practice of neoliberalism as part of the heartland imaginary. Meanwhile, those same power brokers increased surveillance, policing, and incarceration of low-income people, people of color, queer folks, and immigrants as punishment for not fulfilling the white heartland imaginary ideals. This chapter explores privacy-infused arguments for additional rights and protection as well as undergirded fights for the observance of existing rights at the local and regional levels in the heartland.

The following sections illuminate a broad landscape of political activism in the heartland and ultimately argue that the strategies deployed in the heartland informed and fueled the national LGBT political agenda and strategies for the remainder of the twentieth century and into the next. The first section examines how individual organizations staked out their political orientation and audience and then unofficially coordinated with one another to create a more holistic regional AIDS response. The organizations presented here offer a glimpse into the diverse deployments of the white heartland imaginary while also illuminating the behind-the-scenes organizing that made the local and regional political landscape more diverse and complex than what would be represented in the national LGBT agenda. The second looks at education efforts in the region, often led by individuals rather than organizations, with each positioning itself as slightly different than the white heartland imaginary. Interestingly, though not surprisingly within the confines of the white heartland imaginary, most of the people working in the organizations were men, while women dominated the educational spaces, where they often became the spokespersons. The second section explores the particulars of these educators in greater depth, but the gender difference reflects larger white heartland imaginary ideals at work, as women could supposedly disarm, educate, and appear innocent in AIDS educational settings while organizations and the men leading them operated on a different gender landscape within the region. The women examined here all have different proximities to the white heartland imaginary and also to HIV/AIDS, allowing for a better understanding of the nuanced AIDS geography within the heartland. The final section places the heartland regional politics of AIDS in direct conversation with the LGBTQ national political agenda of the last forty years to illustrate the adoptions and failures of heartland strategies at the national level. Together, these sections illuminate the drafting of the blueprint for LGBT politics in the waning years of the twentieth century, showing what became acceptable on the national stage and why, with strategies both limiting and productive.

Political Frames

Missouri's Privacy Rights Education Project (PREP) wrestled with the white heartland imaginary, simultaneously deeply imbricated in its continuation and engaged in struggle against it. As its name suggests, PREP (later PROMO), the political group that ultimately would become the largest political lobbying group on behalf of LGBTQ people in Missouri, claimed LGBTQ and AIDS-related rights through the notion of privacy. Born in the immediate post–*Bowers v. Hardwick* landscape of 1986, when the Supreme Court deemed laws criminalizing sodomy constitutional, the demand for privacy rights by PREP was a thinly veiled demand for gay rights without having to use the words "gay" or "homosexual." Within months of its emergence, PREP also challenged legal attempts and precedents to criminalize persons with HIV/AIDS, whether through incarceration, quarantine, or denial of housing or work protections. As the memory of the *Bowers* decision faded in the larger white heartland imaginary, PREP's focus remained almost exclusively on issues and legislation concerning gay men and lesbians, but their palatability both in lobbying circles and in the wider public increased because of their use of privacy rights as the main framing for their work.

Functionally and materially, PREP was a lobbying group that operated much like most other lobbyists: It made legislative requests, educated the public and legislators with well-tailored spin on potential legislative consequences, worked with legislators to broker compromises and deals, and kept in constant contact with its constituents with frequent small requests. For example, in its January 1995 monthly newsletter, *OUTsmart*, PREP encouraged readers to "Respect Your Elders" by writing a note of protest to President Bill Clinton for having fired US surgeon general Jocelyn Elders.[2] Given the deeply conservative and AIDS-phobic ethos of the 1980s and 1990s

Missouri legislature and governors, which included John Ashcroft, who would become the attorney general for George W. Bush, PREP's impact was surprising. They fought against discrimination in housing based on sexuality and tried to build a community well informed about rights struggles in surrounding states. However, up until autumn 2021, Missouri remained a state where people with HIV faced up to ten to thirty years of imprisonment if they "create a risk of infecting another person . . . with the virus through sex, needle sharing, biting or other established means of transmitting the virus."[3] Discursively, the focus on privacy rights rather than LGBT rights provided a sort of cover for gay rights, almost working as a kind of closet, which allowed PREP to work successfully with more conservative groups and legislators. Here we see a sort of hijacking of white heartland imaginary ideals, individual rights, and privacy to gain access to sites of political power and simultaneously provide discretion to the people PREP represented. This tactical deployment of these ideals translated into the expansion of notions of home to be more (though certainly unreliably and unevenly) welcoming to people with HIV/AIDS and LGBT folks than would have been the case without PREP's small legislative victories. In short, PREP manipulated white heartland imaginary ideals through traditional political routes to fight AIDS and AIDS phobia in the heartland, with mixed results.

Another political frame employed by AIDS activists of the heartland combined political strategies with the assertion of apolitical activism. St. Louis's largest AIDS service organization, St. Louis Effort for AIDS (EFA), first began its work of connecting people with AIDS with additional services in June 1985, but it didn't formally become a 501(c)(3) until the end of that year.[4] By then, it was providing a buffet of services, from support groups to a helpline. In all its services, working above the political fray was a central feature. As one volunteer explained, "Though it had to navigate a very political terrain, it was not political."[5] Of course, AIDS activism was and remains innately political, as is almost everything. Here, EFA relied on its formal 501(c)(3) status, a federal tax status that does not allow political endorsements or speech by the organization, defining politics tightly as related to the electoral realm. By standing technically outside the realm of politics, EFA made great political inroads and progress for people with HIV/AIDS in the heartland region. Although technically it was apolitical, it did not shy away from making people uncomfortable. EFA founder and well-known local drag performer Daniel Flier remembered performing in drag shows and incorporating safe-sex education: "I would unravel condoms out of packages and I'd say, 'This is a condom and this is made of latex and this can save your life.'

I would do this in drag and get right in people's faces and say, 'This goes on your junk before you do anything sexually because if you don't, you die.'"[6]

From its apolitical position, it also created and advocated for services for people with HIV/AIDS. EFA's buddy program paired people living with the disease with volunteers who would check in daily and provide friendship, help with navigating/informing families, and social and emotional support through health crises and end of life.[7] Initially, buddies often lived for only a matter of weeks before succumbing to the disease, but as treatments became available, these relationships lasted longer and services evolved accordingly to provide long-term support, sometimes spread across several EFA volunteers. Additionally, EFA had a helpline and support groups for family members and partners, and it connected people with AIDS with the small number of AIDS-knowledgeable doctors (three or four for the city and surrounding region) and other medical services (often based out of the medical schools at Washington University and St. Louis University). EFA wasn't influencing political campaigns or lobbying for legislation, but it was doing the work of community organizing and service provision on a deeply politicized and stigmatized issue.

Though "apolitical," EFA dominated the AIDS service organization landscape in St. Louis throughout the early epidemic, eventually buttressed by a food outreach organization, PREP, BABAA, DOORWAYS, and many other groups, many of which were started by EFA board members and volunteers.[8] The cross-pollination of board members and activists is critical in understanding the political tactics of the EFA. Publicly embracing the gay community and speaking bluntly and openly about sex epitomized the EFA mission and made open support or financial backing from the state or religious organizations difficult to obtain. Effort for AIDS relied heavily on small grants, volunteer labor, and individual fundraising (until 1988, when it looked to corporations, and then 1990, when the Ryan White CARE Act was passed), at times drawing their entire budget from benefits featuring drag performances.[9] It also made EFA the political foil for other AIDS organizations, which by comparison were almost always more palatable, more respectable, and more closely tied to the white heartland imaginary.[10]

EFA's self-appointed role as the left-anchoring organization of the local AIDS landscape with strong ties in the form of dual board members and volunteers allowed it to serve as a behind-the-scenes political operator of sorts. In the same way that it was not technically political, EFA was not officially involved in the origins of DOORWAYS, the religious interdenominational housing charity for people with HIV/AIDS introduced in chapter 3, but it set the stage for its emergence. With the approval of AZT and other early drugs that granted longer lives to some people, EFA saw the need for housing grow and also saw a potential partner in the city's religious groups, if they were careful to simplify and sanitize the mission. An early DOORWAYS board member and EFA volunteer recalled, "They [religious groups] wouldn't support EFA but they would support DOORWAYS."[11] Thus, when Archbishop May called for compassion for people with AIDS and created an interdenominational working group, inviting an EFA board member to join, EFA had already identified the need for housing, articulated an argument that "housing equals health," and imagined a solution that it simply could not execute without significant resources beyond its means.[12] It was a match made of political strategy or in heaven, depending on one's perspective.

From its inception, DOORWAYS was designed for maximum palatability and highest impact. To accomplish this and foster necessary partnerships with conservative stakeholders, DOORWAYS divorced itself from any services other than housing. Its housing services were very robust and included, from the start, rent subsidies to allow people to remain in the homes they already had and agreements with local landlords to facilitate discounted and subsidized rents, and also construction of homes, ownership plans, and management for those without housing. Today, the organization serves just under 3,000 people in housing that ranges from fully independent apartments to end-of-life care facilities.[13] DOORWAYS did not offer any additional services, for fear of encouraging residents to practice safe sex or "encouraging" homosexuality. Thus, in the interdenominational meetings, EFA and religious leaders envisioned DOORWAYS as devoid of all support services other than housing, with the understanding that EFA could and likely would provide those services separately.[14] Thus, DOORWAYS remained, in the words of one early board member, "vanilla."[15]

In terms of the white heartland imaginary, the examples of PREP, EFA, and DOORWAYS represent three commonly used political framings that ultimately rippled across the country in response to AIDS. EFA presented itself as outside the white heartland imaginary and articulated that position by embracing drag shows, talking openly about sex, and offering services tailored to gay men. Nothing about EFA, aside from its incredibly useful predominant whiteness, suggested at first glance a desire to adhere to or assimilate with white heartland imaginary ideals. Through the cross-pollination of board members and volunteers, along with its position as the first and often the largest local AIDS organization in St. Louis, EFA was able to call on white heartland ideals from other organizations to meet the needs of people with HIV/AIDS when that seemed the best approach. EFA (and specifically its dually appointed board members) did this without losing the capacity to stand outside the bounds of white imaginary ideals, constantly pointing out its harmful consequences. PREP, on the other hand, both deployed and challenged white heartland ideals to access a seat at the policymaking table. Through its use of privacy rights, PREP became legible to both the LGBTQ community and conservative politicians and lobbyists. In both these communities, the concept of privacy rights was highly motivating, but with very distinct meanings for each group. In this way, PREP expanded and protected rights of people with HIV/AIDS by straddling the boundary and meaning of the white heartland imaginary. DOORWAYS, at the other end of the spectrum, was committed and deeply allegiant to white heartland ideals. Palatability, respectability, and religiosity determined the mission, the politics, and the financial resources of DOORWAYS.

These diverse approaches and proximities to the white heartland imaginary are critical to acknowledge and examine as we flesh out the larger history of the early HIV/AIDS epidemic in the United States. Existing literature suggests that LGBTQ politics went the way of DOORWAYS and PREP en masse. In reality, EFA and even ACT UP played critical roles not only in providing the services and political pressures that they did, but also in making PREP and DOORWAYS appear "vanilla" (uncontroversial) and nonconfrontational to white heartland ideals.

The important dynamic shift that occurred at the national level was that board members and volunteers were no longer able to cross-pollinate at the national level, so groups that reimagined home and challenged white heartland ideals (like ACT UP and EFA) had increasingly fewer seats at policymaking tables, while organizations more in line with white heartland ideals were rewarded with access to political power and more robust public support. ACT UP came to play the political foil to the Human Rights Campaign (HRC) and similar organizations on the national scale, and the key difference was that the HRC board and volunteers were almost entirely segregated from the more radical wing of the movement. Furthermore, as the people most excluded by the heartland ideals were among the most creative in reimagining home and challenging the white heartland imaginary, the national focus on more assimilating organizations and aims left them again discursively homeless in the new national LGBTQ political agenda; this was particularly true of communities of color, gender-nonconforming folks, people in poverty, and differently abled people.

Education

Fighting the significant stigma and ignorance surrounding AIDS proved critical to improving the lived experiences of those with HIV/AIDS while also reducing the spread of the disease. Here again, we see different tactics of positioning in relation to white heartland ideals to effectively reach particular audiences. Each of the educators discussed below, much like the political organizations explored above, played a significant role in improving the lives of people with HIV/AIDS in the region and in fighting the spread of AIDS. These educators, like political organizations, deployed a variety of political strategies to gain legitimacy and palatability among intended learners.

Barbara Fassbinder harnessed the power of her position as the embodiment of the white heartland ideal to garner sympathy, to open minds, and to educate others about the risks of HIV/AIDS. Embracing and problematizing the notion of the "innocent victim," much like Ryan White also did to great effect, Fassbinder educated large swaths of the heartland while also fostering real policy changes in the healthcare industry. Fassbinder, a young, religious, white married mother in Iowa, became the first documented case of contracting HIV/AIDS through an accidental needle stick, in the course of her work as an emergency room nurse.[16] Diagnosed in 1986, Fassbinder kept her illness secret until 1990 and then became a national crusader for healthcare precautions against accidental infection and AIDS phobia. Perhaps most famously, she gave testimony in front of the House Subcommittee on Health and Environment in 1991 about occupational safety in the medical field.[17] In her capacity as an outspoken nurse calling for greater regulation, Fassbinder was deeply successful, instituting several new standards around the use of personal protective equipment (PPE) across the medical field. However, she was not simply an advocate for improved labor conditions; she was deeply committed to improving the treatment of people with HIV/AIDS both within and far beyond the medical setting.

Fassbinder's role and success as an educator in the heartland emanated largely from her proximity to both the white heartland ideal and the medical field. When communicating to legislators and lobbying for changes to medical procedures, she foregrounded her experience as a nurse, how she became infected, and the consequences for herself and her family, especially her young children.[18] In speaking with groups ranging from religious organizations to rotary clubs and high schools, Fassbinder often centered her remarks on how she didn't fit the mold of who she thought contracted HIV/AIDS. In positioning herself this way, she effectively communicated to various audiences three important facts central to my argument: first, she was the heartland imaginary ideal in nearly every way; second, if she could get it, anyone could; and third, people with HIV/AIDS should be treated humanely and kindly, in part because she was one of them. This framing amplified her voice in that she could speak as an "innocent victim," in the same way that Ryan White appealed to the larger American public after he contracted HIV during a blood transfusion to treat his hemophilia. Neither Fassbinder nor White accepted the trope of innocent people with AIDS versus guilty people with AIDS, but they both knew they were perceived that way by the white heartland imaginary, and they utilized their positions to educate those in power and the larger public, improve the lived reality of those with HIV/AIDS, and blunt the worst of the AIDS phobia and bias.[19] In this way, they redeployed the white heartland imaginary to fight HIV/AIDS.

Wichita-based AIDS doctor Donna Sweet similarly drew on her white heartland bona fides and her medical expertise to educate the public and those in power to improve the lives of people with AIDS. As she says, "I did a lot of talking to the lay population about this disease, and to their credit, they were just petrified that this was going to be something that if you picked up the telephone after somebody with AIDS had used it that you were suddenly going to have AIDS."[20] She saw her patients being "treated abysmally" and saw the work of educating the communities they lived in as an extension of her care. However, she also drew some important distinctions from Fassbinder and White. Like Fassbinder, Sweet used her positionality to gain entry to and assume importance in educational spaces related to her work, educating against AIDS phobia to improve the lives of her patients. As a straight married woman with deep family roots in Kansas and fluency in the languages of farming, religion, and practicality, she presented the case for HIV education with disarming authority, as wholly unobjectionable yet incredibly effective. Between 1984 and 1994 she gave over 300 AIDS-related talks to lay audiences and another 500 to professional audiences.[21] As a doctor working in a medical school, she also published widely both in medical journals and in the regional press to help educate Kansans about HIV transmission and dispel stigma. However, she went beyond what her credentials as a medical doctor or as a straight white heartland dweller afforded her, leveraging those qualifications into more policy-driven and political spaces.

Understanding the importance of education to prevention, Sweet worked closely with the Kansas Board of Education to ensure Kansas youth of all ages were getting high-quality sex education and HIV-related information in schools. Sweet was invited to the first and only Kansas Governor's

Task Force on AIDS in 1987, and as a result of this "we got mandatory sex education in the school system, and then you fast forward to '97 . . . [when] they did away with universal [sex education] and became district-determined, and about half of the school districts in Kansas went to abstinence-only."[22] The Summer of Mercy in 1991, when thousands of anti-abortion activists affiliated with Operation Rescue National (ORN) protested extensively and dramatically in Wichita and other areas of Kansas, recast the debate about heartland and home and pushed Sweet's safe-sex education focus to the peripheries as abstinence-only education became more politically palatable. While the debates about abortion and AIDS in the 1980s and 1990s were largely distinct from each other, the sudden political push toward abstinence-based sexual education had sweeping implications for both issues in Kansas, the larger region, and eventually the nation, as abstinence-only education spread. Within the span of just a few years, Kansas was transformed from one of the easier states in which to get abortion services to one of the hardest, and Sweet went from being at the head of the table for sexual education curriculum planning to being physically barred from the room by protesters.[23] When the state refused to shift its universal sex education curriculum to abstinence-only in the mid-1990s, right-wing legislators circumvented it by granting individual districts the right to craft their own curriculum, and much of Sweet's work was lost.

The Summer of Mercy was specifically about abortion access, but it spoke the politics of the heartland imaginary and renegotiated definitions of home. Here, in very visible and vociferous ways, members of Operation Rescue rearticulated the religiously and politically conservative understandings of the white heartland imaginary while demanding that women take individual responsibility for pregnancies and adhere to the white heartland ideals of family, religion, and self-sufficiency. This framing dovetailed nicely with the increasingly neoliberal tone of national politics. The Summer of Mercy had a very chilling effect on AIDS education as well, and Dr. Sweet, who had been so successful at leveraging her claim to the white heartland imaginary in her early activism to improve safe-sex education at the state level, suddenly found herself no longer able to claim inclusion in the white heartland imaginary in the same way. Discursively, Operation Rescue had pushed Sweet from her home, from her claim of embodying the heartland imaginary, not by directly attacking Sweet, but by reasserting and redefining the heartland imaginary. As a result, abstinence-only education became ubiquitous, and Sweet's safe-sex educational approach was relegated to speaking engagements and workshops, though she did workshops in more than half of the state's counties.[24]

Just as she did by becoming a primary and secondary curriculum development partner, Sweet continued to expand her expertise in other avenues, even as the route into the public education system evaporated. As her colleagues on the coasts celebrated the passing of the Ryan White CARE Act in 1990 as a welcome, if long overdue, comprehensive AIDS funding legislative package, Sweet realized it was also written with the white heartland imaginary ideals that both dehumanized people with HIV/AIDS and discursively and practically denied them the possibility of existence in the heartland. On average, currently, 150 people per year are newly diagnosed with HIV/AIDS in Kansas. The wording "newly diagnosed in Kansas" is crucial to the history of the medical response, as federal funding offered by the Ryan White CARE Act was calculated and disseminated to states based on the number of newly diagnosed cases, but a significant number of the HIV/AIDS cases in Kansas and other heartland states transferred from coastal states as gay men came home. Sweet explained it clearly: "It was the total number of people diagnosed within your jurisdiction, not per year, but just total diagnosed, so that this large base in New York and California led to very much inequitable care because there was a whole lot more money per person, dollars per person per year if you happened to live in California or New York and needed help than there was in Kansas."[25] As a result, heartland AIDS responders were forced to care for more people per federal dollar. Other federal agencies like the FDA used similar equations that disadvantaged rural states to determine access to drug trials and drug subsidies. The assumption that people infected with AIDS stayed in the place they were diagnosed reflects assumptions about the physical abilities of people with HIV but also reflects the widespread belief that the white heartland imaginary protected the heartland from those infected with HIV by making them invisible and unwelcome. This reality transformed Dr. Sweet into a legislative, lobbying, and fundraising force to meet the needs of her patients and make sure they got equitable access to federal programs.[26] "We had the patients but it didn't look like it according to the way the data was crunched. So we got a little bit of the formula changed. . . . That's how I got started with the lobbying and the national stuff."[27] She became a regular presence at numerous congressional committee hearings at both the state and national levels.

Although both Sweet and Fassbinder tried to keep their activism above the scrum of electoral politics, Sweet's approach to politics differs from Fassbinder's in several ways. First, Sweet was an HIV/AIDS care provider rather than a person infected with HIV, so she had a different positionality to both the epidemic and the white heartland ideals of health and care. Second, she leveraged her white heartland ideals and areas of expertise to expand her politics beyond just the medical and AIDS-education realms. She created angles to work with the Kansas Department of Education and manifested her way into meetings at the White House and on Capitol Hill as an expert on AIDS with legislative acumen. Sweet's work exemplifies a straddling and expanding of the white heartland imaginary, pushing its borders from within to extend them in ways that would improve the lives of people with AIDS.

In sharp contrast, Carole laFavor intentionally worked outside the white heartland imaginary, acknowledging and engaging other understandings of home, medicine, and education. A butch lesbian two-spirited nurse, novelist, mother, and member of the Ojibwe nation, laFavor was diagnosed with HIV in 1986 and quickly became a leading activist in supporting Native Americans with HIV/AIDS. By the time of her diagnosis, she was already a well-seasoned activist for Native American rights, particularly their intersections with violence, women, and queerness. Battling the AIDS epidemic within the Native populations was in many ways a natural progression of this activism.

LaFavor's work garnered her access to some very particular positions of power within the heartland imaginary, such as being featured with a picture and a quote in the 1988 CDC "Understanding AIDS" mass mailing that anchored the America Responds to AIDS campaign, the largest mass mailing campaign in the history of the CDC. Credited simply as Carole, she is quoted in the brochure as saying, "Obviously women can get AIDS. I'm here to witness to that. AIDS is not a 'we,' 'they' disease, it's an 'us' disease."[28] She also sat on the President's Advisory Council for HIV/AIDS, organized by the Clinton administration in 1995.[29] Both of these efforts were directed at increasing HIV/AIDS awareness and prevention in the nation, often echoing the white heartland ideals in numerous ways. In both of these spaces, her identity as a Native woman with HIV/AIDS was foregrounded while her lesbian and two-spirit identities were often unacknowledged, as was the fact that she had contracted HIV through IV drug use.[30] Lisa Tatonetti, who has written extensively on laFavor, writes, "Notably, though laFavor contracted the disease through intravenous drug use and was also an out Indigenous lesbian, the CDC campaign references neither. This decision was undoubtedly part of the CDC's conscious attempt to revise the prevailing public opinion that AIDS was a 'plague' visited on homosexuals and drug users."[31] I would go one step further and suggest that these careful omissions illuminate the ways that those outside the white heartland imaginary were portrayed by the government back to the larger nation, doing the work of crafting the white heartland imaginary narrative in which people of color, Native people, and queer people, when they were acknowledged, were whitewashed, tokenized, and marginalized.[32]

Although she was made somewhat legible to the white heartland through these governmental roles, laFavor dedicated the vast bulk of her energy and activism to speaking to those denied by the white heartland imaginary, and to Native peoples specifically. She founded, co-founded, or led several Native AIDS organizations, including Spirits Alive, Positively Native, and the Minnesota American Indian AIDS Task Force. In each of these venues, she embraced her exclusion from the white heartland imaginary and furthered it by being vocal about her mode of transmission, her lesbian identity, her two-spirit identity, and her experience of sexual violence as important pieces of her personal story and for her Indigenous AIDS activism. While centering all aspects of her identity, she also illuminated the intersections of settler ideologies, white supremacy, patriarchy, homophobia, capitalism, and violence with the spread of HIV/AIDS among Native populations. She effectively used her personal story as an educational tool for Indigenous people and as proof of the web of oppressions that combined with HIV/AIDS to threaten Native communities.[33]

LaFavor firmly rooted herself not only outside of but also in opposition to the white heartland imaginary in several ways. First, she embraced storytelling and the use of films as an important tool for educating Native populations specifically, in keeping with cultural oral traditions. Several of her lectures and interviews were recorded as she made dozens of appearances across Minnesota, North Dakota, South Dakota, and Kansas.[34] She also was the focus of *Her Giveaway*, a 1988 film by Mona Smith, in which she spoke of her experiences living with HIV/AIDS; it was one of the most significant and widely disseminated HIV educational tools by and for Native communities in the world. This was the first of several films in this genre designed to educate Native nations and communities about HIV/AIDS. As a writer, laFavor also interwove Native faith concepts and medicine to make her experiences with HIV/AIDS as a queer Native woman more relatable and understandable to her intended audience, as she also did with her essays and poetry. She advocated for the integration of white and Native medicines in response to AIDS, placing equal value on them. LaFavor also called for universal healthcare, standing in stark opposition to the capital-driven and neoliberalism-celebrating US healthcare system, and pointed out the failings of white medicine in meeting the needs of Native peoples.

Perhaps most compellingly, laFavor called for "health sovereignty," which is emblematic of not only a rejection of the white heartland imaginary but also a reclamation and reimagining of home. Health sovereignty included culturally specific HIV/AIDS programs for Native communities and advocated the use of Native American medical traditions in concert with white medicine to meet the needs of Native people with HIV/AIDS. Along with other Native AIDS activists, including Sharon Day, laFavor turned to Native traditions like medicine wheels and ritual ceremonies, and broader conversations about sexualities and addictions within Native populations to fight the pandemic.[35]

While the integration of culturally specific tools to address health needs within specific cultures is frequently deployed by public health workers and activists working with marginalized communities, I want to examine the concept of sovereignty more, particularly looking at how it is in conversation with the white heartland imaginary and discursive renderings of home. The white heartland imaginary hinges on false assertions of virgin land, white destiny, and resolved land disputes. Native sovereignty emerges as the stark reminder of the truth that reveals the heartland to be a false construction built on exploitation, theft, and large-scale violence against Native peoples. The idea of Native sovereignty, let alone the activism to manifest it, disrupts the white heartland imaginary, first by asserting that Native nations exist in the heartland, then by illuminating the failures of the white heartland imaginary to meet the needs of Native peoples, and finally by rearticulating a space and identity for Native peoples despite the erasing effects of the white heartland imaginary. Sovereignty is at once a reclaiming of a home already in existence, and in terms of AIDS activism, an imagining of a future home, complete with culturally relevant care.

By invoking the concept of health sovereignty amid wider critiques of settler ideologies, homophobia, violence, capitalism, and patriarchy, laFavor effectively portrayed the AIDS epidemic among Indigenous groups as yet another symptom of larger structural illnesses, failures, and violence perpetrated by white society and the white heartland imaginary specifically. Here we see laFavor distancing herself from the white heartland imaginary to effectively communicate with, support, and educate those most intensely ignored and erased by it. While Sweet and Fassbinder leveraged their proximity to the white heartland imaginary to further the fight against AIDS in the heartland, laFavor did the opposite. She could have followed the example set by the CDC and shied away from all her identities, but she recognized that doing so would only further the violent work of the white heartland imaginary as deployed by the forces wanting to erase Indigenous nations and identities.

Heartland Ideals in National LGTBQ Politics

Tactics of straddling heartland ideals took center stage and played a driving role in LGBTQ politics in the final two decades of the twentieth century at the national level. Once deployed by the rising New Right of the 1970s and 1980s, galvanized by the Reagan administration's rhetoric and policies, and demonstrated in action by films, media, and music, the white heartland imaginary became the dominant political narrative of the country, and all political efforts were compared and contrasted with it, regardless of their geographic location. While AIDS itself conflicted with the white heartland imaginary ideals for multiple reasons (its associations with sexuality, drug use, and illness, its health inequities, the racial and sexual communities most impacted—all topics intentionally neglected by the white heartland imaginary), the pandemic demanded a response, leaving activists to navigate a political landscape in which white heartland imaginary ideals dominated.

Heartland activists across the AIDS political spectrum, from those aligned with white heartland ideals to those in direct conflict with them, learned how to redeploy the white heartland imaginary to fight the AIDS epidemic. They carefully orchestrated collaboration across multiple organizations that shared individual board members and activists by design to play out a "bad cop/good cop" or "adhering to/dismantling the white heartland imaginary" dynamic, playing organizations' aims and politics off of each other to produce a meaningful regional AIDS response. We see this in the rise of DOORWAYS and the behind-the-scenes work of EFA. We see this in the extremist light cast on the very small and short-lived ACT UP chapters in the region, which allowed the likes of EFA and health sovereignty efforts to make real progress in the region. Sweet and Fassbinder emerge not only as important activists but also as providing enough white heartland imaginary legitimacy to allow a more robust political and medical AIDS response in the region. The demise of BABAA and its reincarnation within Williams and Associates show the repercussions of pushing against the white heartland ideals too hard and the tactics deployed to circumvent the backlash. The heartland reveals an intricate, innovative, and strategic AIDS response that the larger LGBTQ movement attempted to emulate in its national political agenda in the final decades of the twentieth century and the first quarter of the twenty-first.

While the heartland AIDS response created a sort of safety screen of white heartland assimilation behind which more radical groups and activists could operate and build a more robust AIDS response, the implementation of this strategy at the national scale did not play out the same way. The push for same-sex marriage and the rise of homonationalism exemplify this embracing of heartland ideals in the national LGBTQ political movement. In opting for this approach, political strategists, activists, and organizations orchestrating the national political strategy once again chose a path in which rights have more meaning than justice, in effect cementing the structural inequalities on which rights fall unevenly. Unlike the regional and local activists of the heartland I have discussed, those pushing for same-sex marriage at the national level were myopically focused on that issue and unconcerned with coordinating with other political aims within the LGBTQ movement. There was little strategizing or behind-the-scenes maneuvering to coordinate gains in marriage equality with other rights such as employment rights or housing protections.

Scholars like George Chauncey have already made clear the political rationale for this approach and the relationship between the AIDS crisis and the political push for same-sex marriage.[36] Marriage was a single legal vehicle that could provide nearly all the rights people with HIV/AIDS needed with respect to medical visitation, power of attorney, access to spousal health insurance, inheritance, and taxes, for example. The political calculus of the time figured that a successful (if prolonged) fight for same-sex marriage would be more effective than several individual fights for each right gained through marriage, even if each fight might be less encumbered by the religious pushback on the expansion of legal marriage.

In addition to offering access to a nice package of rights through a simple (if difficult to obtain) political objective, marriage as a goal spotlighted white heartland imaginary ideals and placed them firmly at the heart of the national LGBTQ political agenda. The creation of a family through marriage is the basis of neoliberal governing and economics; in the absence of state services, the successful family can self-sustain. By foregrounding calls for access to marriage, the LGBTQ political agenda effectively communicated to the state and larger society that the majority of LGBTQ people for whom they spoke wanted access to this centerpiece of the white heartland imaginary, challenging it only as much as their inclusion required. The push for same-sex marriage also redeployed the centrality of privacy in LGBTQ rights, not unlike what PREP did in its formation. The issue exemplified the way in which privacy became the contested terrain of LGBTQ rights in the last several decades of the larger political movement. The intensive focus on marriage, the portrayal of often wealthy, white, and cisgendered lesbian or gay couples, and the need to eschew nearly every other issue marginalizing or disadvantaging LGBTQ people (or put distance between them and the marriage goal) all converged to employ the LGBTQ political movement in the sustaining work of the white heartland imaginary and neoliberalism. This came at the cost of LGBTQ issues and activism that questioned or came into conflict with the white heartland imaginary—issues like youth homelessness, HIV/AIDS, job and housing discrimination, and health disparities, to name just a few. These issues did not rely on privacy claims. Instead, they demanded a state or structural response, placing them firmly out of step with the dominant focus on privacy and the self-sustaining, family-focused, and normalizing tactics of the national movement. To be clear, these issues didn't disappear, nor did the activism around them. With the national focus on marriage, these other issues were set firmly to the side and the back by large LGBTQ national lobbying groups that had the money and political power to do so. If the biggest political goal was to gain access to an institution that underpins the white heartland imaginary and neoliberal ideals, then sharing the political stage with issues that pointed out the failures of the white heartland imaginary and demanded a rethinking of social structures made no political sense.

However, even for those who wanted access to marriage, this deployment of the white heartland imaginary in the fight for it didn't align with their motivations. The national battle for same-sex marriage divorced religion from the legal contract and rights of marriage. The heartland regional politics around marriage were framed much differently and reflected, again, a deeper and more complex relationship to the heartland white imaginary ideals. In the heartland, the fight for marriage equality predated the AIDS epidemic significantly and grew from LGBTQ members of religious communities seeking a religious acknowledgment and celebration of their unions. Trinity Episcopal Church of St. Louis began offering home blessings for gay and lesbian couples in the early 1960s to meet this need, and it would eventually provide same-sex unions long before the national Episcopalian leaders or the Supreme Court condoned the practice.[37] In these ways, the heartland's push for same-sex marriage had a different positionality to white heartland ideals than the national campaign did. Religion and religious belief proved to be a major catalyst for marriage equality in the heartland region. In a country awash in white heartland imaginary ideals, that relationship to faith matters. Heartland activists were seeking religious validation and celebration, while national activists were cleaving religion from legal marriage in the hopes of placating religious objections. Thus, even as both the regional and national fought for marriage equality, they did so from very different positions and relationships to white heartland ideals.

Not surprisingly, the move to embrace white heartland imaginary ideals in the marriage fight disproportionately and negatively impacted access to political power, rights, and justice for those in LGBTQ communities who did not adhere to the white heartland ideal: people of color, differently abled people, youths, substance users, gender-nonconforming folks, polyamorous people, and others. Not only were the political issues most salient to these groups effectively sidelined, but they became the foil that made the pursuit of same-sex marriage wholesome, "vanilla," and in line with white heartland ideals.[38] Discussions about youths forced from family homes, violence against trans people, and similar issues that acknowledged that at least some LGBTQ people lived beyond the bounds of the white heartland imaginary largely evaporated from the national conversation on LGBTQ issues and rights and were relegated to smaller organizations like Queer Nation.[39] Another way to understand this division is to return to the notion of privacy. In the introduction to this chapter I summed up the heartland calculus and understanding of privacy: If a person is self-sustaining, which is made significantly easier by whiteness and other structural privileges, they deserve privacy; if they are reliant on the state or larger community, they are justifiably surveilled and denied privacy. Marriage was and is a right that typically facilitates and amplifies self-sufficiency, or at least sufficiency at the family unit level, and thus it is in line with the neoliberal project of off-loading state services onto individuals and families. However, many of the other issues LGBTQ people face demand either state involvement or structural responses, placing them firmly beyond the understood bounds of privacy and, thus, the white heartland imaginary.

In the larger LGBTQ movement, inclusion of the people and the issues that did not align with privacy and heartland ideals became a bargaining chip in the battle for marriage or other rights that were in alignment. A clear example of this political calculus is the bargaining away of the inclusion of trans people in the Employment Non-Discrimination Act of 2007.[40] Meanwhile, the largest national LGBT lobbying groups focused their attention on marriage access and the right to serve in the military, both issues that align closely with white heartland imaginary ideals. In the process of separating LGBTQ issues palatable to heartland ideals from those considered beyond the pale, the most influential national LGBTQ political organizations splintered the communities they claimed to represent, forcing many to question their place in a movement they had believed would offer them a sense of "home," or at least hope for it.[41]

Conclusion

Looking at these heartland examples demonstrates that activism that challenged the white heartland imaginary and neoliberalism existed and thrived in the region. Part of their political power and relevance relied on their ability to infiltrate multiple organizations and coordinate between AIDS organizations and LGBTQ organizations across the political spectrum. This ability dissipated at the national level, such that challenging voices had fewer access points to groups setting the agenda. This also, not inadvertently, led to the quieting of the louder critics of the white heartland imaginary, especially among people of color, gender-nonconforming folks, differently abled people, people with fewer financial resources, and those experiencing housing or financial precarity. Thus, the dominant LGBTQ political narrative and agenda—namely, the fights for marriage equality and the ability to serve in the military—echoed white heartland ideals both in their aims and in who was most vocally fighting for them.

Describing the LGBTQ activism of the late twentieth century as a drift to the center, "intentional abandonment," or assimilationist is both correct and itself a rearticulation of the white heartland imaginary. On the one hand, LGBTQ people and their dominant politics are imbricated in the creation and perpetuation of white heartland ideals that do the work of erasure—particularly the erasure of people of color, Native peoples, disabled people, and the poor, even those who identify as LBGTQ. It is a continued ignoring of the work of people of color, Indigenous folks, trans individuals, and poor people. Similarly, portraying the white heartland imaginary as the opposite of LGBTQ communities denies the existence of religious queers. If we look for those voices, which are muffled by the roar of the white heartland imaginary, we will find a much more nuanced, vibrant, politically diverse, and healthy politics undergirding LGBTQ political activism, particularly at the local and regional levels in the late twentieth century and now.

Conclusion
Expanding Outward

On April 14, 2022, Democratic Missouri state representative Ian Mackey spoke directly to Republican representative Stephen Basye, who had introduced a legislative amendment that would ban transgender high school students from participating in athletics:

> MACKEY: I remember that you said . . . that your mother called you to tell you that your brother had some news that he was afraid to tell you.
>
> BASYE: Okay.
>
> MACKEY: And your brother wanted to tell you that he was gay, didn't he?
>
> BASYE: Um, he was, uh, expressing that to the family, and he thought that uh, that we would hold that against him and not let my children be around him.
>
> MACKEY: Why do you think he thought that?
>
> BASYE: Uh, I don't know. It never would've happened, I can tell you that. My kids, at that point in their life, adored my brother.
>
> MACKEY: Can I tell you, if I were your brother, I would have been afraid to tell you, too. I would've been afraid to tell you, too. Because of stuff like this. Because this is what you're focused on. This is the legislation you want to put forward. This is what consumes your time. I would've been afraid to tell you, too. I was afraid of people like you growing up, and I grew up in Hickory County, Missouri. I grew up in a school district that would vote tomorrow to put this in place. And for eighteen years, I walked around with nice people like you who took me to ball games, who told me how smart I was, and who went to the ballot and voted for crap like this. And I couldn't wait to get out. I couldn't wait to move to a part of our state that would reject this stuff in a minute. I couldn't wait, and thank God I made it. Thank God I made it! And I think every day of the kids who are still there who haven't made it out, who haven't escaped from this kind of bigotry. Gentlemen, I am not afraid of

you anymore because you are going to lose! You may win this today, but are going to lose.¹

A video of the two-minute dressing down traveled beyond the usual reach of Missouri state legislative deliberations, attracting the attention of National Public Radio, CNN, and other national news outlets. The exchange, in which a standing and sonorous Mackey passionately attacked Basye (who is well known for his bluster and insult-filled social media posts and speeches) as he sat quietly, almost ashamedly, stood in stark contrast to the tidal wave of anti-LGBTQ and specifically anti-trans bills that saturated the 2022 and 2023 legislative seasons in states as far-flung as Florida, Idaho, Arizona and Missouri. As the number of such bills over these two years rose past 500, Mackey's speech appeared as a bright spot despite its futility in opposing the legislation.² A version of Missouri House Bill 2140 went on to pass in June 2023, along with dozens of other bills across the country that limited access to gender-appropriate bathrooms, healthcare, athletics, and legal name and gender marker changes, especially for youths.

The Mackey-Basye exchange captured the essence of how the battles over home, the articulations of the white heartland imaginary, and the concept of privacy that sculpted the heartland AIDS response continue to structure the political horizons years later. In his excoriation of the legislation, Mackey offers three visions of home, each a deeply contested space: the one of his youth, in which he felt discursively homeless; the one of the material district that he currently represented, which would "reject this stuff a minute"; and the one in the future for which he is fighting (both discursively and materially), which has far murkier borders. He is following in the footsteps of other Missourians like the Trinity Episcopal Church priest Bill Chapman, who tried to call on the better angels of the populace to point out bigotry and offer up a more compassionate response. In a longer comment on social media, Basye's response ended with, "It didn't phase me at all, I went home afterwards, enjoyed a delicious glass of Maker's 46 Bourbon, then laid down and slept like a baby!!"³ Deceptively simple, the rejoinder evokes the image of a man with nothing on his conscience, enjoying a singularly American liquor in its most rugged form—another invocation of the heartland imaginary echoed throughout this book.

The last decade has given a national microphone and an adrenalin shot to two dueling versions of a white heartland imaginary. Both contain characteristics of the white heartland imaginary that shaped the AIDS response. Both claim to reflect the soul of the nation, a stand-in for the heartland. For example, in an impromptu courthouse speech immediately following his conviction for thirty-four felonies, President Trump declared, "It's OK, I'm fighting for our country. I am fighting for our constitution."[4] On one hand, there is the heartland ideal built on whiteness, heteronormativity, gender binaries, and neoliberalism. We can trace this in the rhetoric of the MAGA political movement, the recent deluge of anti-trans legislation in dozens of states across the country, the thinly veiled racism of anti-wokeness and anti-immigration stances, and the scramble for control over local school boards and state curriculums. The constant needling of "the coastal elite" does the work of claiming the heartland as the physical site of home and belonging for this worldview. In his memoir, *The Courage to Be Free: Florida's Blueprint for America's Revival*, Florida governor Ron DeSantis offers a master class in deploying a very specific version of the heartland that includes Florida, demonstrating that the heartland has little geographical meaning.[5] First, he makes clear what the heartland is *not* by pointing to the "elites" who demarcate the coasts (though here again, the geographic location of these elites matters less than their politics and beliefs that mark them as "coastal"). A *Washington Post* review of the book pointed out the heavy lifting "elites" do in the book's introduction, which attacks "America's 'elites,' in all their various forms—'progressive elites,' 'woke elites,' 'public health elites,' the 'scientific-technological elite,' 'bureaucratic elites' and 'power-hungry elites.' The word 'elite' gets used more than 20 times in the book's introduction, which is 12 pages long."[6] From there, he goes on to ground himself in the heartland through his upbringing by "gritty, working-class, God-fearing" parents from Pennsylvania and Ohio and casting himself as the ostracized nonelite during his time at Yale University (for his undergraduate degree) and Harvard Law School. Here, the division is the point, creating a strong sense of belonging and home for those who meet the ideals, and ostracism, mocking, and threats for those who do not. From this division and rhetoric grows devotion and fervor from those who belong, and precarity and discursive and material homelessness for those who do not.

On the other hand, there is a white heartland imaginary, largely formulated during the Obama presidency, in which capitalism (or, in some cases, neoliberalism) offers a new chance at equity or "a fair shake," compassion, and tolerance (to a degree). We can track the careful crafting of this version of the white heartland imaginary in the immediate governmental response to the economic recession of 2008 in the form of a massive bailout of US automakers that undergirds the image of the factory-working Midwesterner and the heartland pickup truck.[7] Obama singing "Amazing Grace" in a church ravaged by violence evoked a comfort, humility, and religious ethos that resonates with the version of the heartland he deployed throughout his time in office, even as he sang from a lectern in South Carolina. The rainbow of color reflecting off the White House edifice the night the Supreme Court ruled in favor of marriage equality was a literal projection of the tolerance that is one of the two central components of this version of the heartland. The other element, capitalism, appears in the intense leveraging of capitalist ideals (competition and market prices) in the negotiated Affordable Care Act (Obamacare) and climate legislation. Even as many of these signature moments occurred outside the physical heartland region, they sculpted the "soul of the nation," for which the heartland remains a proxy.[8]

As I write this in the waning days of the 2024 election, we see these dueling heartland imaginaries articulated in particularly strident ways as Trump promises to "Make America Great Again" (again connoting a coda to an earlier historical time) and Harris offers "A New Way Forward." An "angry" Trump is juxtaposed with a "joyful" Harris; the intense focus on immigrants as threats to physical and financial (and even family pet) security versus a concentration on having "far more in common than we have that separates us" fuels endless pre-election commentary. These themes are simply articulations of the past several presidential cycles and seemingly the only options our current national political discourse makes possible.

The heartland as an imagined future is not only rhetorically crafted by these campaigns but also populated by the archetypes of the heartland each presidential candidate has conjured with their vice presidential running mate. The fact that each candidate chose a running mate from the geographic region of the heartland speaks to its continued importance in our national identity. The primary reason Trump and Harris chose J. D. Vance and Tim Walz, respectively, was to harness the power of the heartland imaginary to mobilize voters. These two vice presidential candidates accentuate both the similarities and the already stark contrasts in the two versions of the heartland on offer this election cycle. Both are straight white men, married with children, with military backgrounds, modest origins, and, apparently, a shared love of Diet Mountain Dew, but the similarities seem to end there. Even these few basic shared facts illuminate a great deal of the overlaps in the two versions of the heartland in this contest. The whiteness, maleness, straightness, working-class roots, and association with the military (a proxy for patriotism) echo the rough outlines of the white heartland imaginary articulated in the 1980s. Even as one of the presidential candidates is a Black and South Asian woman from San Francisco, her vice presidential candidate Tim Walz has brought a heartland sensibility to the campaign, signified by camouflage campaign gear, well-worn flannel shirts, deployments of "common sense," football analogies, and devotion for the Minnesota State Fair (the "big get together," as locals call it). Meanwhile, J. D. Vance has been introduced as Trump's political heir apparent, but from Ohio and with a book (*Hillbilly Elegy*) turned movie about growing up and out of the heartland. Both men, though opposite in many ways, are meant to represent, embody, and reflect the heartland, only making more obvious its imagined and sculpted discursive boundaries. As we experience these two imaginary heartlands battling one another, much can be gleaned by asking who is denied access to the imagined ideal, to the home each politician declares is the real United States. Who is erased in these articulations, and why? With this question, we quickly realize that these two versions of the heartland are insufficient.

Both these iterations of the heartland imaginary are limited; they are functionally two sides of the same coin, despite their cosmetic (though real policy) differences. Both are hemmed in by their reliance on large state institutions designed to foster stability, not justice; a shared and deeply flawed history of exceptionalism and meritocracy; and an economic system that rewards exploitation and greed. While one version is certainly safer precarity than the other for LGBTQ folks, people of color, those with different abilities, and those experiencing economic and housing, neither offers a clear pathway to true liberation or "home" for them. They both continue to render many people discursively and materially homeless. The Obama, Biden, and now Harris version of the heartland keeps issues of gender, sexuality, and health separate from economics and the environment by focusing on tolerance on the one hand and economics on the other. At times, there is an attempt to combine these issues, as in the stimulus package passed amid the COVID-19 pandemic that sought to target financial aid and resources to specific disadvantaged groups, from childcare workers to incarcerated people.[9] However, the legislative process almost always rendered these attempts futile, as such provisions were traded away for votes for the legislation.[10] In this way, this version of the heartland imaginary is not dissimilar to the 1980s version that anchored non-Southern whiteness, heteronormativity, and economic independence. Tolerance is certainly better than hate, but it is a far cry from nurturing (discursive and material) home for everyone, and it isn't meeting the moment of today. We see this in action when Ian Mackey offers only the hope that "you are going to lose," without revealing how.[11] In these ways, these white heartland imaginaries of today are clear descendants of the version of the 1980s.

Fortunately, even as these two versions of the heartland imaginary dominate the national discourse, they are not the only versions. Just as we see in

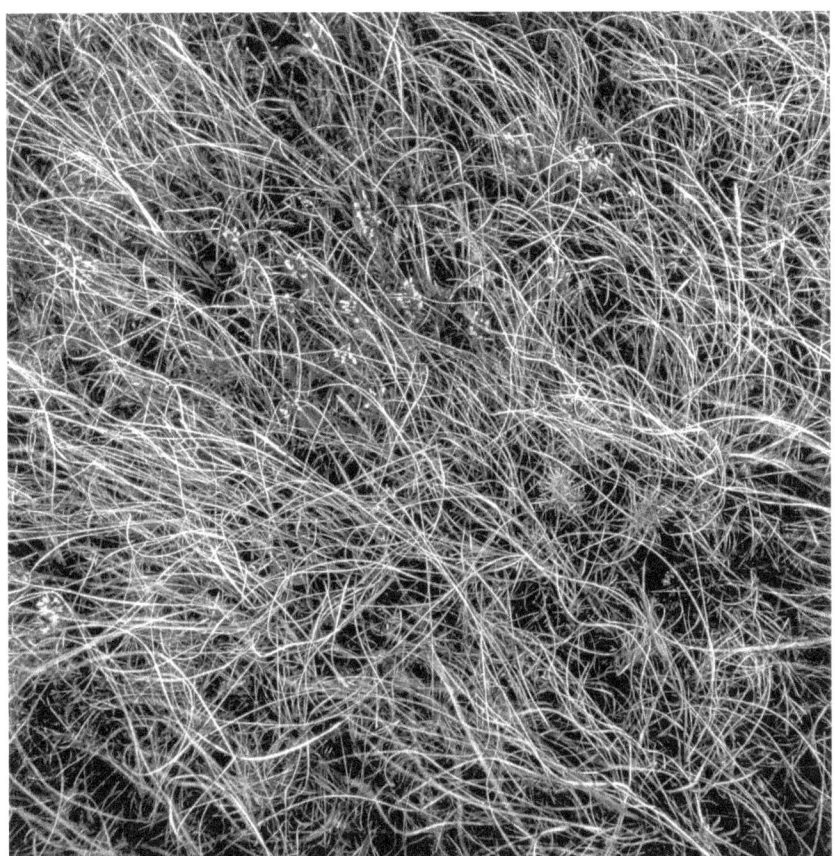

FIGURE C.1 Terry Evans, *Fent's Prairie, Salina, Kansas, 1978*. Spencer Museum of Art, University of Kansas, Gift of Terry Evans, 1980.0147.

the heartland AIDS response (really, in the history of any marginalized group), a reimagining of the heartland (beyond the white imaginary) and discursive home can and does occur despite an exclusionary or oppressive white heartland imaginary. These alternative articulations emanate from a centering of oppressed groups and prove far more expansive in their analysis and liberatory in their potential. Theorists, particularly Black feminists, Latinx and Chicana feminists, and trans and queer theorists, have provided a rich and diverse analysis on navigating new types of home under systemic oppression and discrimination.[12] Such reimaginings don't happen in statehouses or courtrooms, but amid the tangle of the grasses at our feet at the beginning of this book (figures C.1 and 1.3).

Today, there are several examples of such alternative homes and heartlands, just as there were in the history of the early AIDS crisis in this region. The Black Lives Matter (BLM) movement emerged in July 2013 in the aftermath of the acquittal of George Zimmerman in the 2012 shooting death of seventeen-year-old Trayvon Martin, but it took full form not far from where several groups and people in this book originate.[13] Even in its own telling of its history, the organization makes clear that "the Black Lives Matter Global Network would not be recognized worldwide if it weren't for the folks in St. Louis and Ferguson who put their bodies on the line day in and day out, and who continue to show up for Black lives."[14] Just fifteen miles north of St. Louis sits Ferguson, Missouri, and though BLM is often positioned as part of the coastal elite and conceptualized as a movement anchored by the coasts, it is, in fact, deeply Midwestern, intertwined with the heartland and simultaneously imagining a new heartland. Here, the death of Michael Brown in 2014 at the hands of local police sparked mass protests.[15] From these protests arose a clear mission "to eradicate white supremacy and build local power to intervene in violence inflicted on Black communities by the state and vigilantes. By combating and countering acts of violence, creating space for Black imagination and innovation, and centering Black joy, we are winning immediate improvements in our lives."[16] Led by queer women Alicia Garza, Patrisse Cullors, and Opal Tometi, this movement centers imagination, innovation, and joy and demands a reimagining of a heartland in which people of color could be at home. This requires massive overhauls of not just racial hierarchies and police but also the economic system that hinges on carceral systems that produce profit off of mass incarceration, healthcare systems that ensure illness for the poor through high costs, lack of access, and medical research that centers whiteness, heterosexuality, and cis men. The 2016 police killings of Philando Castile in Minneapolis and Alton Sterling in Baton Rouge added greater fuel and urgency to the call for structural change, showcasing how people of color are often denied the comfort and protection of home, belonging, and right to life in public spaces. In 2020, the death of George Floyd in Minneapolis, Minnesota, brought into stark clarity the unlivable realities of those rendered discursively homeless as a video recording of his killing depicted Floyd using his final breaths to repeatedly plead, "I can't breathe."[17] Though his words were meant literally, as police officers pushed the life out of him with the weight of their oppressive bodies, they also resonate figuratively as he was denied the freedoms of home, the most basic of which is the ability to breathe and live. The Black Lives Matter movement offers a vision of home and the heartland that is much broader than the limited versions constructed by the main political parties. Here, home expands far beyond mere tolerance in which simple survival in a violent system signals success, to include a more capacious and liberatory future that promises thriving and creating with the help, rather than hindrance, of large systems and communities.[18]

While it may seem a leap from the early AIDS response of the 1980s, the loss of life at the hands of oppressive state structures and lack of care resonates and certainly links these histories. Similar too is the diversity of activism and the necessity to think expansively about the complexity of the issues at work. Certainly, the most dramatic and large-scale ACT UP protests offer images of streets and public places filled with protesters that are similar to those of Black Lives Matter marches and protests around the world. The use of religious infrastructure to provide AIDS services and support also displays reimaginings of old systems that echo much of what BLM articulates as goals.

Mutual aid responses offer a similarly expansive vision of home and the heartland. The early months of the COVID-19 epidemic saw one of the largest-scale implementations of mutual aid in modern times, precipitated by the unprecedented and abrupt interruption of capitalism on many fronts. With the near-global economic shutdown after the immediate arrival of COVID-19, much of the neoliberal emphasis on individual bootstrapping and self-sustainability as the only path to true success became temporarily destabilized, if not replaced, by an emphasis on caring for community. En masse, we got to know our neighbors in new ways through toilet paper sharing, new food systems, impromptu childcare solutions, and creative community care for the sick and differently abled, all amid constantly changing restrictions and limitations. We connected to and supported each other socially, financially, and medically through watching online drag shows and concerts, buying local, and wearing masks.[19] Although the financial precarity created by capitalism is typically shamed and hidden, COVID illuminated in a sympathetic spotlight just how many individuals and families experience food insecurity, how many small businesses live on the edge of financial ruin, and how many communities depend on state services ranging from public schools to public health.[20] The essential workers who are regularly undervalued by the economy and society literally had people across the nation banging pots and applauding every night in their honor during the early months of the pandemic.

For those few months, the heartland expanded to new extents, centering those typically on the peripheries (from the sick to the economically precarious). This expansion was doubled by the contemporaneous Black Lives Matter protests and the time and attention society at large had to watch, engage with each other, and contemplate these overlapping pandemics of COVID-19, racism, and capitalist exploitation. For many, this new reality that prioritized community and care over individuals and shame felt new, but communities seen as outside the heartland or discursively homeless (or at least precarious) have been using mutual aid for decades and continued to do so during and after COVID lockdown. Consider the massive carpooling network of the Birmingham bus boycott, attempts to house and feed immigrant and refugee populations, and community supports for trans and queer youth. These are all communities whom capitalism and the state are designed to marginalize and disempower, for whom home is precarious at best, and who are rarely claimed as part of the heartland. These are also communities that regularly deploy mutual aid as a critical tactic for survival.

The early AIDS response in the heartland and beyond hinged on mutual aid, whether through volunteer-run organizations like the Gay Men's Health Crisis in New York, St. Louis's EFA, or the nun-run hospice in Wichita. Care for community and not just the individual is the backbone of HIV/AIDS activism and services. Considering the early COVID response alongside the early AIDS response provides a striking contrast that showcases the depth of the stigma of AIDS, the intensity of state apathy, and the isolation experienced by people with AIDS. In the early months of COVID, the state, which for the last several decades has shrunk and qualified its public services, suddenly used its power to pause evictions, offer free medical care for all, and infuse billions of dollars into public education and health, local governments and businesses, and individuals. Here, the state amplified, celebrated, and nurtured mutual aid efforts to the extent that only the state could. An equally robust state response to AIDS comparable to that of COVID would have required far less in terms of money, disruption, and implementation (medical research, safe-sex education, employment protections, a pause on evictions of those with HIV/AIDS, free condoms, and needle exchanges). Yet, the political appetite and social pressure for such interventions simply didn't exist, because of perceptions of who was getting the disease and the modes of transmission. In the absence of the state, mutual aid met as many needs as it could. It still does for those living with AIDS in the heartland today, and increasingly so as Medicaid qualifications are further limiting and benefits diminish under state regulations. Through creative community responses, mutual aid has always done the work of approximating home for those rendered precarious or discursively homeless, offering another vision of the heartland in which interdependence is not only accepted but celebrated as a source of communal strength.

Indigenous anti-pipeline activism offers yet another expansive version of the heartland in which the earth itself becomes a key figure in understandings of home, heartland, and community. Led by trans and two-spirited people, this movement demands that the land and waterways be protected from oil pipelines that hurt the world not only by fostering burning fossil fuels but also by leeching and leaking into soil and waterways. The Standing Rock protests of 2016, in which the Standing Rock Sioux tribe in North Dakota protested the construction of the Dakota Access pipeline, is the best-known recent example of this activism, but the tradition of Native peoples protecting the earth from colonizing and capitalist extractive forces is rich and long.[21] With the national press given to the Standing Rock protest, the role of two-spirit and queer folks was highlighted, with one organizer, Big Wind, saying, "The majority of people at [the protesters'] camp are queer. Nearly half use gender pronouns. Behind the scenes, there are so many queer people up here in the North fighting this pipeline who understand the intersectionality between the oppression that we all face as BIPOC [Black, Indigenous, and people of color] queer people." Making the connection between queerness, home, and pipeline activism, Big Wind went on to explain, "There are pipeliners on Grindr trying to find people to hook up with. So it's men and queer people, too, who are dealing with this extractive economy. When we talk about the abuse that's done to the land and to Indigenous people, they go hand in hand at the end of the day. They see us as inferior, and they see the land as a commodity. That's their perception. The violence that's done against us and the violence against the Earth are connected."[22]

Within the movement, the heartland and home expand to include the intricate connection between humanity and the earth while illuminating the costs of capitalism and fossil fuel reliance on the land, on society, on Native communities, and on individual bodies.[23] This construction of heartland and home gains strength and urgency amid the global climate crisis. With increasingly intense tornadoes, storms, heat, and drought, the heartland as a geographic region is seeing people become instantly, literally, and materially homeless as a result of violent storms and flooding while simultaneously facing existential climate realities. This expansive construction of the heartland and home, as inextricably linked to the health of the earth and its people, will become increasingly vital to future survival.

The meta-scale and multivalent framing of this existential threat at the heart of Indigenous anti-pipeline activism resonates with the emphasis on humanity at the center of the heartland AIDS response. Both movements underline a commonality to unite people while also having a clear sense of the various tendrils of oppression and inequality at play. While the anti-pipeline activism hinges on the health of the earth and its implications for larger humanity, the early AIDS response emphasized the shared humanity of those with HIV/AIDS and those not infected. This notion of shared humanity spurred much of the religious and medical activism in the region, which in turn created services and additional spaces to meet the needs of those most oppressed and precarious in the AIDS epidemic. Much like two-spirit, lesbian activist Carole laFavor in the heartland AIDS response, many of the activists driving the anti-pipeline work make clear connections between the colonial and capitalist roots of their physical realities and discursive precarity. This ability to draw clear lines between exploitative structures, personal suffering, and the commonalities of humanity propel both movements.

The Black Lives Matter movement, the growth of mutual aid, and the two-spirit-led Indigenous anti-pipeline movement showcase new formations of discursive homes, imagined futures, and redistributions of social values that open the door of possibility and reality for less violent and more fairly allocated material homes. In doing so, they offer new constructions of the heartland. Each of these movements is rhetorically and culturally excised from the heartland, but they are here. Harnessing new and evolving technology like social media to share these discursive homes on an unprecedented scale, these movements emerge quickly and speak loudly. These are examples of those willing to imagine a different world, unafraid (or perhaps just alienated enough) to abandon the flawed current structures and systems in search of something better. They echo and rhyme with the creativity and passion of the early AIDS response in the heartland that drew on healthcare delivery by way of crop duster, EFA education efforts, and even the short-lived heartland ACT-UP. In this current reaching and dreaming and struggle, we again witness the unlikely collaborations, the behind-the-scenes strategizing that allow for those most erased to gain purchase, voice, and representation that epitomized the heartland AIDS response. Efforts to replace broken structures, build and rely on interdependent communities, and see beyond the trappings of wealth and political power to see the precarity and potential of humanity reverberate across all these movements. Through these lenses, a new home emerges, and the heartland remains amorphous but infinitely flexible to include us all. This contestation and (re)imagination of home and the constant (re)construction of the heartland lies at the center of the history of not just the heartland AIDS response but also so many of the movements and politics that define our present and shape our future.

Acknowledgments

This book wouldn't have been possible without those who lived this history. I wish that AIDS had never happened and that no one had to experience the suffering, tragedy, and rage it has caused for nearly half a century. But those who did experience the darkest, early years have been an incredible source of inspiration, pushing me along in this project, even as the weight of this history became almost too heavy at times. Those who died from AIDS and/or red tape in this era stirred outrage and grief that motivated me to tell this history. Equally pivotal in the manifestation of this book were those who survived, those who provided care, those who organized, and those who bore witness to this history. I want to thank all of those who have taken time to share their personal experiences with me through oral histories and personal archives, and also the literally dozens of people who would informally share their experiences of the pandemic over the grocery checkout, at the cocktail party, or at the community pool. One of the most striking aspects of writing this book was that it truly seemed to give almost everyone I spoke with an opportunity to share a story. The sheer volume of these interactions demanded that I take on this project.

In addition to the interactions with neighbors, the archives of this region are bursting with untold stories of HIV/AIDS. The librarians, archivists, and research assistants who helped me plumb the archive proved invaluable, as always, in bringing this history back to life. Tami Albin helped me plot and correct my course several times in meeting rooms in the library with whiteboards and legal pads, over email, and, by the end, perhaps by osmosis. Her research and oral history project, Under the Rainbow, was a treasure trove of sources as well as a useful provider of context. Stuart Hinds, the curator of the amazing Gay and Lesbian Archives of Middle America (GLAMA), took special care to pull incredible collections and introduce me to many figures who proved important in understanding this history, including Austin Williams, to whom I am also indebted for his vast knowledge of the Kansas City AIDS experience. Who knew that when I met a fellow graduate student fifteen years ago, he would later be the lynchpin of historical and archival knowledge for my work? Such was the case with Ian Darnell, who opened the doors and archives of St. Louis for me. Student research assistants Korbin Painter and Matthew Cannedy also provided much help in processing oral interviews and identifying potential archives.

I was afforded the time to research and write this book by a summer stipend from the National Endowment for the Humanities, a full fellowship from the American Council of Learned Societies, a Franklin Research Grant from the American Philosophical Society, two semester-long Hall Center Research Fellowships, two awards from the General Research Fund at the University of Kansas, and a semester-long sabbatical. Having the time and ability to focus my attention on this research and writing has been a gift without which this book would have suffered greatly. I especially want to thank Kathy Porsch for teaching me how to write grants.

One of the greatest strengths of the University of Kansas is its people, especially my colleagues in women, gender, and sexuality studies. I enjoy being in conversation with all of them and appreciate the engagement with my work through the Hall Center Gender Seminar, as well as less formal chats in the office or over beers. Special thanks to Stacey Vanderhurst, Aimee Wilson, Nick Syrett, Sarah Deer, Abe Weil, Marta Vicente, Akiko Takeyama, Alesha Doan, Hannah Britton, Ayesha Hardison, Jeanne Vaccaro, and Krystofer Meadows. It is truly a joy to work alongside such incredible colleagues, all in one department. The Hall Center for the Humanities at the University of Kansas has not only provided me with fellowships but also several spaces in which to share my work, get wonderful feedback, and exchange ideas across the university. Thank you to Giselle Anatol and Andrew Hodgson for making the Hall Center what it is.

Beyond the University of Kansas, there is the vibrant field of the history of sexuality and the history of AIDS specifically that helped nurture this book in one way or another. Specifically, I would like to thank Margot Canaday, Reg Kunzel, Marc Stein, Julio Capo Jr., Darius Bost, Dan Royles, Jonathan Bell, LaShonda Mims, Stephen Vider, Kevin Murphy, Don Romesberg, and Sarah Schulman for engaging with, shaping, and inspiring my research and writing. There are a handful of scholars whose feedback brought this manuscript into its final form, making it much stronger in many ways. The Burn It All Down writing group consisting of Nic John Ramos, Emily Hobson, Salonee Bhaman, Myrl Beam read several versions of much of this manuscript and truly helped me and propelled me to transform it from a thin, jumbled set of ideas into the book it has become.

Andreína Fernández, an editor at The University of North Carolina Press, shepherded and nurtured this book along for several years. Her enthusiasm never wavered, even at times when the book needed a lot of work. Most importantly, she found the absolute best reviewers for this manuscript who helped bring it to its potential: Anthony Petro and Emily Hobson. Anthony Petro gifted tremendous insight and thoughtful comments that strengthened the book, especially in thinking through and clarifying the sections on religion. Emily Hobson gave thoughtful reviews both as she read my work in our writing group and also as an anonymous reviewer for the press. In these two roles, she alone has grappled and engaged with this work more than anyone else. Emily is truly a treasure of our field, a generous thinker, a provocative scholar, and an all-around good person. I am thankful to the entire team at The University of North Carolina Press, where my experience has been smooth, professional, and top-notch. Additionally, I want to express deep gratitude for the incredible work of Mary Ann Lieser, indexer extraordinaire.

Mentors have buoyed me throughout my professional life. François Furstenberg taught me to love the craft of history, especially the importance of oral history to the subjects I care most deeply about. John D'Emilio and Jennie Brier not only guided me through graduate school successfully but have remained steady and constant touchstones to whom I can return, often unannounced, to find a warm welcome and sage advice. Having them both always in my corner is a great privilege and gift. At the University of Kansas, Alesha Doan and Nick Syrett have been most influential in shaping my professional career as a delicate balancing act between life, research, teaching, and service.

An amazing small cadre of brilliant scholars, who I also count among my closest friends, served the unique role of both guiding me (sometimes dragging me) through the research and writing process while also serving as confidants, comics, and just the right balance of co-conspirators and taskmasters. Emily LaBarbera-Twarog, Myrl Beam, and Jessica Gerschultz, thank you! In many ways, this project was born out of a walk in the prairie with Jess—thanks for telling me it was an interesting idea worth exploring more. Emily, Myrl, and Jess each brought different eyes and ears to this project, but more importantly, they provided the deep friendship forged through almost daily phone calls that sustain me as a human and encourage me to find balance between work and life. Natalie Cisneros, with whom I talk less frequently but connect with no less deeply, has also been a source of strength and joy, all while also serving as an academic sounding board. The research and writing of this book overlapped with COVID, the death of my stepmom, becoming chair, and several other challenges. They pulled me through it all. Without them I would be far less happy, productive, and balanced, and likely would be lost out in a field or on a bike trail somewhere, terrified of snakes.

While I love my research and job, those friends who are entirely removed from it keep me grounded, laughing, and able to put myself and my work into a much larger perspective. Henry Schneiderman, Chrissy Torrey, Rémy Lequesne, Lydia Lequesne, Nicole Reiz, Emily Ryan, Jeff Colosino, Aaron Glazer, Zoe Fraade-Blanar, the staff and teachers of Cordley Elementary, the Wednesday night tennis lesson crew, and the random Sunday afternoon game gang, thank you for bringing so much life and joy into my life, not to mention support. Our relationships, all unique, sustain me in a way that few others do.

My chosen and biological families are the ones who made this book possible. Over my entire life, they have shaped who I am and what I study. They have always had my back, even when we didn't agree, and cheered me on even when they didn't understand the goals I was attempting. My mom, Jane Callahan-Moore, and my dad, John Batza, instilled in me resilience, strength, patience, curiosity, and a strong, unwavering belief that I am loved and I am capable. These attributes, along with the excellent education they made sure I received, have proven the bedrock of my career and to my approach to life. Karyn Batza, who passed away during the writing of this book, reinforced these gifts from my parents, and I am forever grateful that she was my stepmom. Her final gift to me was a renewed and deeper bond with my step- and half-siblings Ricci, Jeff, and Kim. My sister Jen has, at various times in my life, been my hero, my tormentor, my comrade in arms, but most of all, one of my very best friends, with whom I can always find a way to laugh even when things are hard and dark. I am so thankful I have gotten to share my life with her by my side from the jump. My aunt Pattie, along with Uncle Mike, have been constant cheerleaders as well as a reliable source of good conversation and laughter. My aunt Maggie Calloway, who passed away in November of 2024, remains truly inspirational in her resilience, kindness, curiosity, and perseverance in the face of unbelievable odds. My uncle Danny, both Aunt Barbaras, and Barbara Sue round out my Batza/Moore family choir of support and inspiration who leave me humbled and thankful. I also consider myself endlessly lucky in that I am an honorary member of the Magnuson family. Bobbie, Rod Jr., Sue, Jamie,

Lindsay, Kylie, and Nick, thank you for your friendship and love over the last twenty-something years! Stephanie Swann has provided a steady, bright guiding light, a North Star in my sky, for over thirty years. I am so grateful to have found her, Nancy, and all of their critters.

Lastly, I want to thank Kellie and Elliot, who have had to live with this book for several years now but have always cheered me on, even though we were all sick of it by the end. Elliot continues to amaze me every day, as he has since he was born. Watching him grow up is the greatest gift, and chatting with him about politics, global news, comedy improv, and whatever else he's into in any given moment is always one of the brightest parts of my day. After more than twenty years, Kellie continues to grow with me, push me to be a better person, and love me completely on good days and bad. She is life's very best dance partner, and I thank her for being exactly who she is and for how she shows up in the world every day.

Notes

Introduction

1. Erika Mills, "June 5, 1981—The First Report of AIDS in the U.S.," Circulating Now, National Library, National Institutes of Health, June 4, 2021, https://circulatingnow.nlm.nih.gov/2021/06/04/june-5-1981-the-first-report-of-aids-in-the-u-s/.
2. Mayor's Task Force on AIDS, "Recommendations of the Education Committee: Gay and Bisexual Men," October 1987, MS 180, Box 1, Folder 2, Steven R. Pierce Collection, Gay & Lesbian Archive of Mid-America, University of Missouri–Kansas City (hereafter cited as GLAMA).
3. Bailey, *Sex in the Heartland*.
4. Erise Williams, interview by Katie Batza, May 31, 2018.
5. Daniel Flier, interview by Katie Batza, January 10, 2019.
6. Sister Joann Stuever, interview by Katie Batza, February 6, 2019.
7. Chuck Gulas, interview by Katie Batza, December 14, 2018.
8. We can also trace these factors in the Black and Native response to race-driven neoliberal attacks.

Chapter One

1. Hamer, "Abandoned in the Heartland."
2. I am also drawing on Higby, "Heartland."
3. Baum, *Wonderful Wizard of Oz*; *The Wizard of Oz*, directed by Victor Fleming (Los Angeles: MGM, 1939; Burbank, CA: Warner Home Video, 2005).
4. Other scholars have offered up concepts that also resonate with my approach to the heartland. Halberstam, *In a Queer Time*; Bey, *Cistem Failure*; Ahmed, *Strange Encounters*.
5. Manalansan, Nadeau, Rodríguez, and Somerville, "Queering the Middle."
6. Schulman, *Seventies*.
7. *Footloose*, directed by Herbert Ross (Los Angeles: Paramount, 1984).
8. Much theoretical work exists on the role of the nation as a political and rhetorical formation, as well as the role of the state in controlling bodies. I would begin with Benedict Anderson, Michel Foucault, Frantz Fanon, Stuart Hall, Marita Sturken, and David Morley. Anderson, *Imagined Communities*; Foucault, *Discipline and Punish*; Sturken, *Tangled Memories*; Morley, *Home Territories*; Hall, *Essential Essays*.
9. Frank, *What's the Matter with Kansas?*
10. Frank labels those beyond the cover of the white heartland imaginary with the term "liberal" and traces how liberals become both generally villainized and blamed for all sorts of political, economic, and social problems in Kansas. For the purposes of

this book, I look beyond electoral politics and the increasing divide between Red America and Blue America.

11. Thrasher, *Viral Underclass*; Esparza, "Black Bodies on Lockdown"; Sophie Hurwitz, "After 30 Years, Missouri Reforms HIV Transmission Criminalization Law," *Missouri Independent*, August 5, 2021, https://missouriindependent.com/2021/08/05/after-30-years-missouri-reforms-hiv-transmission-criminalization-law/.

12. Ehrman, *Eighties*; Hayward, *Age of Reagan*; Johnson, *Sleepwalking through History*; Perlstein, *Reaganland*; Frank, *What's the Matter with Kansas?* This farming reality was ushered in with the 1973 Farm Bill, signed into law with great fanfare by President Nixon.

13. Darman, *Landslide*.

14. Morrison, "Home."

15. Davenport, "All This"; Hoganson, *Heartland*.

16. For more on the urban rural divide even within the heartland region, see Herring's *Another Country*.

17. United States Bureau of the Census, *1990 Census of Population and Housing*, https://www2.census.gov/library/publications/decennial/1990/cph-2/cph-2-27.pdf.

18. Fink, *Meatpacking Line*; Nabhan-Warren, *Meatpacking America*; Warren, *Great Packing Machine*.

19. Deer, *Beginning and End of Rape*; Griffith, *Words Have a Past*; Krupat, *Changed Forever*.

20. Hoganson, *Heartland*; Branham et al., *Quantrill's Raid*; Connelley, *Quantrill and the Border Wars*.

21. Tricia Masenthin, "Marker Dedication Pays Tribute to 3 Black Men Lynched 140 Years Ago in Lawrence," *Lawrence Times*, June 10, 2022, https://lawrencekstimes.com/2022/06/10/marker-dedication-pays-tribute/; Krehbiel, *Tulsa, 1921*.

22. US National Park Service, "Kansas," https://www.nps.gov/nico/index.htm.

23. Office of Public Affairs, US Department of Justice, "Three Southwest Kansas Men Sentenced to Prison for Plotting to Bomb Somali Immigrants in Kansas City," press release, January 25, 2019, https://www.justice.gov/archives/opa/pr/three-southwest-kansas-men-sentenced-prison-plotting-bomb-somali-immigrants-garden-city.

24. Halvorson and Reno, *Imagining the Heartland*.

25. Herring, "'Hixploitation' Cinema"; Cartwright, *Peculiar Places*.

26. "AIDS Comes to a Small Town," Oprah.com, November 16, 1987, www.oprah.com/oprahshow/aids-comes-to-a-small-town/all#:~:text=In%20July%201987%2C%20the%20tiny,in%20the%20local%20swimming%20pool.

27. Shilts, *And the Band Played On*.

28. Carroll, *Mobilizing New York*; Schulman, *Let the Record Show*; Bost, *Evidence of Being*; Royles, *Make the Wounded Whole*; Cohen, *Boundaries of Blackness*; Bhaman, "Few Months of Peace"; Brier, *Infectious Ideas*; Brier, "Locating Lesbian and Feminist Responses"; Bell et al., "Interchange"; Ramos, "Poor Influences"; Mumford, *Not Straight, Not White*; Petro, *Wrath of God*.

29. Cartwright, *Peculiar Places*.

30. Larry Kramer, "1,112 and Counting," *New York Native*, March 14–27, 1983; San Francisco AIDS Foundation, "Resource," https://www.sfaf.org/resource-library/sfaf-history/.

31. "Robert Rayford," National Park Service, accessed October 28, 2024, www.nps.gov/people/robert-rayford.htm.

32. Ayala and Spieldenner, "HIV Is a Story"; Rea Carey and Jesse Milan Jr., "The Whitewashed History of HIV," Plus, June 14, 2018, https://www.hivplusmag.com/stigma/2018/6/14/whitewashed-history-hiv-black-teen-died-aids-1969.

33. Steve Hendrix, "Mystery Illness Killed Boy, Years Later Doctors Learned What It Was," *Washington Post*, May 15, 2019, https://www.washingtonpost.com/history/2019/05/15/mystery-illness-killed-boy-years-later-doctors-learned-what-it-was-aids/. Tissue samples had been stored in a research laboratory at Tulane University in New Orleans.

34. Centers for Disease Control, "Pneumocystis Pneumonia—Los Angeles 1981," *Morbidity and Mortality Weekly Report* 30, no. 21 (June 5, 1981): 250–52.

35. Department of Public Health, Bureau of HIV, STD, and Hepatitis, HIV/AIDS Surveillance Program, "HIV Statistics 2011–2020," https://www.legis.iowa.gov/docs/publications/FCTA/1220262.pdf.

36. McKay, *Patient Zero*; Pépin, *Origins of AIDS*.

37. Carey and Milan, "Whitewashed History of HIV"; Gina Kolata, "Boy's 1969 Death Suggests AIDS Invaded U.S. Several Times," *New York Times*, October 28, 1987, A15; John Crewdson, "Case Shakes Theories of AIDS Origin," *Chicago Tribune*, October 25, 1987, www.chicagotribune.com/news/ct-xpm-1987-10-25-8703200167-story.html.

38. "Community AIDS Update Statistical Report," MS 180, Box 2, Folder 2: MTF-AIDS Community AIDS Update, Steven R. Pierce Collection, GLAMA.

39. "Community AIDS Update," MS 180, Box 2, Folder 2: MTF-AIDS Community AIDS Update, vol. 1, no. 1, p. 2, May–June 1987, Steven R. Pierce Collection, GLAMA; HIV Epidemiology and Field Services, *AIDS in New York City, 1981–2007* (New York: Department of Health and Mental Hygiene, March 2009); Carey and Milan, "Whitewashed History of HIV."

40. Herring, *Another Country*; D'Emilio, "Capitalism and Gay Identity." For example, Iowa did not track and report to the CDC HIV infections—just AIDS cases and deaths—throughout the entirety of the pre-HAART era.

41. The coming home syndrome would prove incredibly important in both the politics and medical realities of people with HIV.AIDS in the heartland. It will be discussed in much more depth in future chapters. "Community AIDS Update."

42. "HIV News and Statistical Report," KCMO Health Department—HIV/AIDS Program, 1993, Steven Pierce Collection, Box 3, Folder 8, University of Missouri Kansas City, Kansas City, Missouri.

43. Jay Johnson, interview by Katie Batza, May 9, 2017; Donna Sweet, interview by Katie Batza, February 5, 2019; Sheryl Kelly, interview by Katie Batza, March 7, 2019; Vernon, *Killing Us Quietly*.

Chapter Two

1. Capozzola, "Very American Epidemic"; Hobson, "AIDS Quilt in Prison"; Testa, "'If You Are Reading."

2. To be clear, to be discursively homeless means to be unbelonging in and unwanted by the larger region and nation for which it serves as an imagined white ideal

of home. Being materially homeless refers to a physical break with a previously established home; this can sometimes overlap with being unhoused, but not necessarily.

3. Hall, *Essential Essays*, 362.

4. Hammonds, "Missing Persons."

5. Crimp, *Melancholia and Moralism*; Crimp and Bersani, *AIDS*.

6. Davenport, "All This," 89.

7. Moraga and Anzaldúa, *This Bridge Called My Back*; Anzaldúa and Keating, *This Bridge We Call Home*; Lugones, *Pilgrimages/Peregrinajes*.

8. Anzaldúa and Keating, *This Bridge We Call Home*, 3.

9. Anderson, *Imagined Communities*.

10. Vider, *Queerness of Home*, 3.

11. Foucault, *Discipline and Punish*.

12. Donna Sweet, interview by Katie Batza, February 5, 2019.

13. Jay Johnson, interview by Katie Batza, May 9, 2017.

14. J. Johnson, interview.

15. J. Johnson, interview.

16. J. Johnson, interview.

17. J. Johnson, interview; "Ahalya Project Providing Assistance to HIV-Infected Native Americans in OKC, Tulsa," Native Health Database, accessed on October 28, 2024, https://nativehealthdatabase.net/digital-heritage/ahalya-project-providing-assistance-hiv-infected-native-americans-okc-tulsa.

18. In fact, even finding statistics for HIV/AIDS infection for Native Nations and people can still be challenging, as the Centers for Disease Control still organizes much of its data by categories that do not include Native peoples. However, recent studies show that some Native communities have an infection rate nearly double that of white people. "HIV/AIDS and American Indians/Alaska Natives," Office of Minority Health, Department of Health and Human Services, accessed on May 6, 2024, https://minorityhealth.hhs.gov/hivaids-and-american-indiansalaska-natives.

19. Centers for Disease Control, "Recommendations of the U.S. Public Health Service Task Force on the Use of Zidovudine to Reduce Perinatal Transmission of Human Immunodeficiency Virus," *Morbidity and Mortality Weekly Report* 43, 1994, accessed on April 16, 2025, https://www.cdc.gov/mmwr/preview/mmwrhtml/00032271.htm.

20. Evelyn Cohen, interview by Katie Batza, November 1, 2018; Chuck Gulas, interview by Katie Batza, December 14, 2018; Keith Price, interview by Katie Batza, October 29, 2018.

21. "DOORWAYS Needs Help Furnishing Residences," *Frontline: The Monthly Newsletter of St. Louis Effort for AIDS*, August 1988, Box 1, Folder Newsletters 1988, St. Louis Effort for AIDS Collection, Missouri History Museum (hereafter cited as St. Louis EFA Collection); Gulas, interview.

22. Cohen, interview; Gulas, interview; Opal Jones, interview by Katie Batza, November 30, 2018.

23. Gulas, interview; Michael Allan to John May, "The Doors Are Open Letter," September 14, 1988, Box "Executive," Folder "Archbishop and Bishop—Correspondence—1988–1997," St. Louis Archdiocese Library and Archive, St. Louis

Archdiocese (hereafter cited as St. Louis Archdiocese Library); "Just Months Old, Doorways Becomes a Community and a Place PWAs Call 'Home,'" *Frontline: The Monthly Newsletter of St. Louis Effort for AIDS*, November 1988, Box 1, Folder Newsletters 1988, St. Louis EFA Collection.

24. "Just Months Old."
25. Batza, "Opening DOORWAYS," 229–32.
26. Spade, *Mutual Aid*.
27. Gulas, interview.
28. Halberstam, *Queer Art of Failure*.
29. Herring, *Another Country*; D'Emilio, "Capitalism and Gay Identity."
30. Gulas, interview.
31. Gulas, interview; Gary Hirshberg, interview by Katie Batza, September 26, 2018.
32. Sweet, interview.
33. Esparza, "Great Gay Return: AIDS 'Homecoming' Narratives and Middle America's Fantasies of Racial Reconciliation."
34. Sweet, interview.
35. Sweet, interview.
36. Tom Harper, interview by Katie Batza, October 2, 2018.
37. Gulas, interview.
38. Gulas, interview; Bill LaRock, interview by Katie Batza, July 10, 2018; Cathy Johnson, interview by Katie Batza, July 9, 2018.
39. Forstie, *Queering the Midwest*. *Queering the Midwest* traces LGBTQ communities in supposedly "unfriendly" places, finding that LGBTQ identity is rarely the driving force behind LGBTQ events or organizations; instead, it is a sort of LGBTQ ambivalence that drives a different sort of community formation among LGBTQ folks in the region. While I agree that LGBTQ organizing in the heartland region is substantively different than on the coasts or in big cities, I argue it is less about "ambivalent communities," as Forstie argues, and more about a deep practicality and political acumen to garner necessary services for a small LGBTQ community in a deeply conservative and religious landscape.
40. LaRock, interview.
41. LaRock, interview.
42. LaRock, interview; C. Johnson, interview.
43. LaRock, interview.
44. LaRock, interview.
45. C. Johnson, interview.
46. LaRock, interview.
47. LaRock, interview.
48. Sturken, *Tangled Memories*, 13.
49. "Lesbian Icon Phyllis Lyon Dies at 95," *Windy City Times*, April 15, 2020, 5; "Phyllis Lyon and Del Martin: Beyond the Daughters of Bilitis," *LGBTQ History and Culture since 1940*, Part I, Gale Primary Resources, accessed February 1, 2024; Jones, *When We Rise*.
50. Bey, *Cistem Failure*; Bey, *Them Goon Rules*; Puar, *Terrorist Assemblages*; Puar, *Queer Tourism*; Butler, *Precarious Life*; Butler, *Undoing Gender*; Foucault, *Discipline and Punish*;

Foucault, *Birth of the Clinic*; Foucault, *History of Sexuality*; Halberstam, *Queer Art of Failure*; Halberstam, *In a Queer Time*; Halberstam, *Trans*; Cartwright, *Peculiar Places*.

Chapter Three

1. Keith Price, interview by Katie Batza, October 29, 2019.
2. Petro, *After the Wrath of God*; Carroll, *Mobilizing New York*; Schulman, *Let the Record Show*.
3. Petro, *After the Wrath of God*; O'Loughlin, *Hidden Mercy*; White, *Reforming Sodom*; Cohen, *Boundaries of Blackness*; Royles, *Make the Wounded Whole*.
4. "Shanti Model of Peer Support," Shanti Project, accessed May 15, 2024, www.shanti.org/about-us/shanti-model-of-peer-support/.
5. Moreton, *To Serve God*; Nabhan-Warren, *Meatpacking America*; Curtis, *Muslims of the Heartland*; Wuthnow, *Red State Religion*; White, *Reforming Sodom*; Petro, *After the Wrath of God*.
6. Murray, *Not in This Family*; Petro, *After the Wrath of God*; Rzeznik, "Church and the AIDS Crisis"; Whitney Cox, "Christian, Philadelphian, and Gay-Affirming Responses to AIDS 1982–1992" (PhD diss., Temple University, 2016), Proquest (10144379); Bell, "Between Private and Public"; Kowalewski, *All Things to All People*.
7. Michael Slawin, interview by Katie Batza, June 12, 2018; Chuck Gulas, interview by Katie Batza, Decemeber 14, 2018; Jim Thomas, interview by Katie Batza, August 27, 2018.
8. Gulas, interview.
9. "Modern Mission Jan. 25," *Now*, January 1963; Ian Darnell, "The Gospel of the Gay Ghetto: Neighborhood Churches and Queer Communities in the Era of the Urban Crisis, St. Louis, 1950s–1970s," unpublished manuscript, 22.
10. Darnell, "Gospel of the Gay Ghetto," 23. The Exit was located at the corner of Westminster Place and N. Boyle Avenue. "Political Actions and Organizing: 1945–1992," *Mapping LGBTQ St. Louis*, v1 Esri Story Maps, October 2017, http://wustl.maps.arcgis.com/apps/ MapTour/index.html?appid=1a3bb142caa140018df5dc432a88bc80.
11. "Presenting the Mandrake Society," n.d. [ca. 1969], Box 1, [St. Louis] Lesbian, Gay, Bisexual, and Transgender History Project, sa1038, State Historical Society of Missouri Research Center, St. Louis, Missouri.
12. Humphreys, *Out of the Closets*, 82–83; D'Emilio, *Sexual Politics, Sexual Communities*, 60; Wilson "Seed Time," 36.
13. Humphreys, *Out of the Closets*, 85–89; *Gay St. Louis* 4 (July/August 1978) 15, in collection 545, Folder 267, Western Historical Manuscript Collection, University of Missouri–St. Louis; Police Report, Complaint No. 412758, 1–2, 4; Darnell, "Gospel of the Gay Ghetto," 24; Wilson, "Seed Time," 36.
14. Humphreys, *Out of the Closets*, 90.
15. *Mandrake*, May 1971, 2. Surviving copies of *Mandrake* are archived in the Laud Humphreys Papers, Coll2007-012, ONE National Gay and Lesbian Archives, Los Angeles, CA; Darnell, "Gospel of the Gay Ghetto," 24; Wilson, "Seed Time," 36.
16. For an example of the ad, see *Mandrake*, March 1971.

17. Rodney Wilson, private collection.

18. In the first half of the decade, the congregation elected two openly gay members to the lay leadership board. Ian Darnell, interview with Bill Chapman, July 1, 2013; Ian Darnell, telephone interview with Jim Pfaff, March 25, 2014.

19. *Mandrake*, May 1971; Baker and Taylor, *History of Trinity Church*, 34.

20. Darnell, "Gospel of the Gay Ghetto," 24; "Lent—1976," n.d., Trinity Parish Archives.

21. Hanhardt, *Safe Space*; Miller, "Coalitional Fronting."

22. Miller, "Coalitional Fronting."

23. Perhaps the most obvious example of this intersection is the founding of the Metropolitan Community Church by Troy Perry in 1968.

24. "About Us," St. Louis EFA, accessed May 5, 2019, www.stlefa.org/about_efa.

25. Baker and Taylor, *History of Trinity Church*, 43.

26. These political organizations will be explored in greater depth in chapter 5.

27. Baker and Taylor, *History of Trinity Church*, 43, 46.

28. Jym Andris, email to Katie Batza, July 23, 2018.

29. Jym Andris, interview by Katie Batza, August, 21, 2018; Rodney Wilson, interview by Katie Batza, July 17, 2018; Philip Deitch, interview by Katie Batza, September 12, 2018; Gary Hirshberg, interview by Katie Batza, September 26, 2018.

30. Trinity Episcopal Church Guide to Art and Design Brochure, accessed April 16, 2025, https://www.trinitycwe.org/_files/ugd/4a4931_f64eb92da1974142a7b90e5fbf155076.pdf; Baker and Taylor, *History of Trinity Church*, 35, 39.

31. Baker and Taylor, *History of Trinity Church*, 35.

32. Baker and Taylor, *History of Trinity Church*, 35.

33. Baker and Taylor, *History of Trinity Church*, 35.

34. Lydia Chaves, "Man in the News: John Lawrence May," *New York Times*, November 12, 1986, A28.

35. National Conference of Catholic Bishops, "Statement: The Many Faces of AIDS," United States Catholic Conference, November 14, 1987, www.usccb.org/resources/statement-many-faces-aids-november-14-1987.

36. Ari Goldman, "Catholic Leader Rebuts O'Connor on Condom Issue," *New York Times*, December 30, 1987, A1; "Some Catholic Bishops Say Condom Policy Is 'Mistake,'" *Los Angeles Times*, December 15, 1987.

37. Colman McCarthy, "AIDS, Condoms and the Cardinal's Answer," *Washington Post*, January 10, 1988, H08.

38. Ari Goldman, "Bishops to Reconsider AIDS Paper That Backed Condom Education," *New York Times*, December 29, 1987.

39. "National Conference of Catholic Bishops News Conference," C-SPAN.

40. Minutes of the Ad Hoc Task Force on AIDS, March 6, 1987, Box "Administrative," Folder "Files-RG03C13," St. Louis Archdiocese Library; "Task Force on AIDS to Start Work Here," *St. Louis Review*, April 3, 1987, 1, 7; "Called to Compassion and Responsibility," National Conference of Catholic Bishops and United States Catholic Conference, www.usccb.org/issues-and-action/human-life-and-dignity/global-issues/called-to-compassion-and-responsibility.cfm.

41. "Doorways Announces New President and CEO," *Vital Voice*, accessed May 14, 2024, http://thevitalvoice.com/tag/aids/page/3.

42. Gulas, interview.

43. Evelyn Cohen, interview by Katie Batza, November 1, 2018. Both the Episcopalian communities and the Lutherans also gave regularly, though the amounts often fluctuated. Minutes of the Core Committee of the Catholic Task Force on AIDS, April 25, 1988, Box "Executive," Folder "Archbishop and Bishop—Correspondence—1988," St. Louis Archdiocese Library (hereafter cited as Minutes of the Core Committee). Also, the United Way provided some significant start-up funds. "AIDS Housing Program Gets Strong Start-Up Support," *Frontline: The Monthly Newsletter of St. Louis Effort for AIDS*, February 1988, Box 1, Folder Newsletters 1988, St. Louis EFA Collection.

44. Gulas, interview; Cohen, interview; Minutes of the Core Committee, September 26, 1988; Minutes of the Core Committee, June 27, 1988; Minutes of the Core Committee, April 25, 1988.

45. Cohen, interview.

46. Price, interview; Cohen, interview; Jones, interview; Jim Timmerberg, interview by Katie Batza, Katie Batza, December 6, 2018; "St. Francis Residence Opens Its Doors in Clayton," *Frontline: The Monthly Newsletter of St. Louis Effort for AIDS*, March 1988, Box 1, Folder Newsletters 1988, St. Louis EFA Collection.

47. Cohen, interview; Gulas, interview; Price, interview; Flier, interview; Minutes of the Core Committee, April 25, 1988.

48. Allan to May, "Doors Are Open"; "Just Months Old."

49. Gulas, interview; "Just Months Old."

50. Michelle O'Brien, "Catholic Health Outreach Program Survey on AIDS Response," February 1987, Box "Executive," Folder "Archbishop and Bishop—Correspondence—1987," St. Louis Archdiocese Library.

51. Cohen, *Boundaries of Blackness*; Royles, "Don't We Die, Too?"; Bost, "At the Club"; Levenson, *Secret Epidemic*.

52. Allan to May, "Doors Are Open."

53. Jones, interview; Gulas, interview.

54. This type of collaborative politics is examined in depth in Stewart-Winter, *Queer Clout*.

55. "Readers' Advocate Explains Why Gay Rights Bill Was Not Covered in *Post-Dispatch*," *St. Louis Post-Dispatch*, December 13, 1992, 40; Tim O'Neil, "Revised Gay Rights Code beyond 'Routine,'" *St. Louis Post-Dispatch*, December 13, 1992, 40, 44.

56. Associated Press, "Virtually Unnoted, St. Louis Approves Gay Rights Measure," *New York Times*, December 28, 1992, www.nytimes.com/1992/12/28/us/virtually-unnoted-st-louis-approves-gay-rights-measure.html?fbclid=IwAR2YidDv8oB_RPLcxow_p99Xwi_rEKHG6SAWNdfqSxFFAQWUSGgBNk7g_R4.

57. *The Ordinance Project*, directed by Austin Williams, documentary film, 2018, GLAMA.

58. Gulas, interview; Cohen, interview.

59. Brawley and the St. Louis LGBT History Project, *Images of Gay and Lesbian St. Louis*.

60. Gulas, interview.
61. Wilson, interview; Slawin, interview; Thomas, interview.
62. Mayer and Pat Levy, interview by Katie Batza, December 4, 2018 Gulas, interview; Cohen, interview.
63. Gulas, interview.
64. Gulas, interview.
65. Williams, interview; Gulas, interview.
66. Cohen, interview; Jones, interview; Brenda Armour, interview by Katie Batza, December 11, 2018.
67. Gulas, interview.
68. Levy, interview.
69. Gulas, interview.
70. Levy, interview.
71. Barrett-Fox, *God Hates*.
72. Barrett-Fox, *God Hates*.
73. Williams, *Ordinance Project*.
74. For more on the battle for same-sex marriage rights in Kansas, see Janovy, *No Place like Home*. Since starting research on this book and learning of the ubiquity of Westboro Baptist protests in the heartland, I often ask my classes if anyone has encountered Westboro protests. Without fail, at least 10 percent and as many as half of my students have seen a protest in action, often targeting their high schools for having a LGBTQ student group, a queer homecoming court, or an out member of the school's sports team or musical group. I myself have been the target of protest for giving a lecture on this research—all nearly a decade after Fred Phelps himself has died and the congregation is in decline.
75. Barrett-Fox, *God Hates*.
76. Johnson, interview.
77. Brier, *Infectious Ideas*; Fassbinder, "Time to Face the Enemy"; Herring, "Tribute to Barbara Fassbinder, RN."

Chapter Four

1. J. Johnson, interview.
2. Sweet, interview.
3. Sweet, interview.
4. Sweet, interview.
5. Sweet, interview. Here, "come-homers" are what Dr. Sweet calls those who were diagnosed out of state and then came home for end of life.
6. Sweet, interview.
7. Sweet, interview.
8. Sweet, interview.
9. Sweet, interview; Kelly, interview.
10. Sweet, interview.
11. Sweet, interview.
12. Sweet, interview; Kelly, interview.

13. Kelly, interview.

14. Sweet, interview.

15. Sweet, interview.

16. Now in her seventies, Sweet still works full time but fortunately has two nurse practitioners and a junior colleague who have taken up the work of the clinics outside of Wichita. There are now five full-time people dedicated to the job she once did primarily on her own.

17. Williams, interview.

18. Williams, interview.

19. Williams, interview.

20. Royles, *Make the Wounded Whole*; Cohen, *Boundaries of Blackness*; Bost, *Evidence of Being*.

21. Williams, interview.

22. The Minority AIDS Initiative, an agreement between Clinton and the Black Congressional Caucus, in 1998, 1999, 2000. "Minority AIDS Initiative," Clinton White House, accessed October 10, 2023, https://clintonwhitehouse4.archives.gov/ONAP/cbc/cbc_toc.html.

23. *Tongues Untied*, directed by Marlon Riggs, documentary/experimental film (San Francisco: California Newsreel, 1989).

24. Williams, interview.

25. Williams, interview.

26. Ballroom culture is perhaps most famously explored in the documentary film *Paris Is Burning* and also in the fictionalized television series *Pose*. In ballroom culture, which blends competitive dancing with culture and the making of queer chosen families for predominantly low-income queer men of color since the 1970s and continuing today. Ballroom emerged in New York City among predominantly Black and Latino people ostracized from the lager drag community due to racism and discrimination. During balls, the "families" or "houses" "walk" or face off against one another in a series of categories like realness or vogue or runway in which competitors display their artistry and style for judges.

27. Williams, interview.

28. Williams, interview.

29. Williams, interview.

30. The Minority AIDS Initiative continued through the George W. Bush period, but the Bush administration made it easier for faith-based and predominantly white AIDS organizations who purported to serve minority groups to gain access to the previously protected Minority AIDS Initiative funds.

31. Tim Murphy, "BABAA Black Sheep," *POZ*, accessed April 24, 2023, www.poz.com/article/BABAA-Black-Sheep-545-8776.

32. "St. Louis: AIDS Agency That Hired Porn Star Loses Aid," The Body Pro, November 1, 2002, www.thebodypro.com/article/st-louis-aids-agency-hired-porn-star-loses-aid.

33. Williams, interview.

34. Williams, interview.

35. Stuever, interview.

36. Chinh Doan, "Game-Changer: Nebraska AIDS Project Reacts to UNMC Breakthrough Research," KETV, July 2, 2019, www.ketv.com/article/game-changer-nebraska-aids-project-reacts-to-unmc-breakthrough-research/28270366; Ashly Richardson, "HIV Breakthrough: UNMC Medical Research Results in New Medicine," First Alert 6, June 10, 2022, www.wowt.com/2022/06/09/breakthrough-medical-research-unmc-with-new-hiv-medication/; Jeffrey Robb, "UNMC, Temple Research Increases Chances of Eliminating HIV Infection," University of Nebraska Medical Center, May 2, 2023, www.unmc.edu/newsroom/2023/05/02/unmc-temple-research-increases-chances-of-eliminating-hiv-infection/.

37. Wilson, interview.
38. Wilson, interview.
39. J. Johnson, interview.
40. Stuever, interview.
41. Stuever, interview.
42. Stuever, interview.
43. Stuever, interview.
44. Stuever, interview.
45. Stuever, interview.
46. Stuever, interview.
47. National Conference of Catholic Bishops, "Called to Compassion."
48. Stuever, interview.
49. Stuever, interview.

Chapter Five

1. Gilmore, *Golden Gulag*; Gilmore, *Abolition Geography*.
2. "Respect Your Elders!," *OUTsmart* (St. Louis), January 1995, 1.
3. "What You Need To Know About Missouri Laws On HIV, Missouri Department of Health and Senior Services (2008)," Center for HIV Law and Policy, March 2008, www.hivlawandpolicy.org/resources/what-you-need-know-about-missouri-laws-hiv-missouri-department-health-and-senior-services; Hurwitz, "After 30 Years."
4. "St. Louis Effort for AIDS Fact Sheet," c. 1986, Box 1, Folder Newsletters, Timothy Cusick Collection, Missouri History Museum.
5. Anonymous, interview by Katie Batza.
6. Flier, interview.
7. Levy, interview by Katie Batza; Gulas, interview; Anonymous, interview.
8. Flier, interview.
9. Flier, interview; "Corporate Funding Has $100,000 Goal," *Frontline: The Monthly Newsletter of St. Louis Effort for AIDS*, February 1988, Box 1, Folder Newsletters 1988, St. Louis EFA Collection.
10. The one major exception here is local branches of ACT UP, which were short-lived, especially for St. Louis, in part because all the other local AIDS organizations shunned them for being beyond the pale politically. In fact, in 1991, nearly half of the EFA board of directors resigned when they learned that the EFA offices had been offered as a free meeting space for the local ACT UP chapter; ACT UP found another meeting location.

11. Gulas, interview; Flier, interview. Though this is largely true, there are a few notable exceptions where EFA received grants from religious groups, such as the 1988 grant from St. Luke's Episcopal-Presbyterian Charitable Fund that allowed EFA to hire its first paid staff. "EFA Received $71,500 Grant for Hiring Paid Staff," *Frontline: The Monthly Newsletter of St. Louis Effort for AIDS*, August 1988, Box 1, Folder Newsletters 1988, St. Louis EFA Collection.

12. Gulas, interview; Minutes of the Core Committee, April 25, 1988.

13. DOORWAYS, "Impact Report 2018," factsheet, accessed May 7, 2019, https://doorwayshousing.org/app/uploads/2022/07/FY18-impact-report-final_print_web.pdf.

14. Minutes of the Core Committee, June 27, 1988.

15. Gulas, interview.

16. Herring, "Tribute to Barbara Fassbinder, RN."

17. "Barbara Fassbinder Testimony," Box 1, Barbara Fassbinder Papers, University of Iowa, Iowa City.

18. Fassbinder, "Time to Face the Enemy."

19. Renfro, *Life and Death*.

20. Sweet, interview.

21. Donna Sweet, private collection.

22. Sweet, interview; Kelly, interview.

23. Wichita was home to the Women's Health Care Services, one of only three clinics across the country that provided third trimester abortions. The medical director, George Tiller, became the well-known villain of anti-abortion activists who blocked the entrance to the clinic through sit-ins for the entire summer of 1991, resulting in hundreds of arrests. His clinic was firebombed in 1986 and then rebuilt. In 1993, Tiller was shot five times by an anti-abortion extremist inspired by the recent assassination of another abortion provider. He recovered and continued to offer services. In 2009, George Tiller was assassinated by another anti-abortion extremist, inside a church where he was serving as an usher. Joe Stumpe and Monica Davey, "Abortion Doctor Shot to Death in Kansas Church," *New York Times*, May 5, 2009, www.nytimes.com/2009/06/01/us/01tiller.html.

24. Sweet, interview.

25. Sweet, interview.

26. Joe Stumpe, "The Sweet Spot: Access to Care," KU School of Medicine–Wichita, October 1, 2019, www.kumc.edu/school-of-medicine/campuses/wichita/about/news/news-archive/the-sweet-spot-access-to-care.html.

27. Sweet, interview.

28. *Perspectives in Disease Prevention and Health Promotion* (Centers for Disease Control, 1988).

29. "An Unprecedented Problem: The Clinton Administration and HIV/AIDS in the United States," Clinton Digital Library, accessed October 8, 2023, https://clinton.presidentiallibraries.us/an-unprecedented-problem-the-clinton-administration-and-hiv/aids-in-the-united-states.

30. Davis, "Understanding AIDS"; Montgomery et al., "Health Belief Model"; Centers for Disease Control, "Perspectives in Disease Prevention and Health Promotion

Understanding AIDS: An Information Brochure Being Mailed to All U.S. Households," *Morbidity and Mortality Weekly Report* 37, no. 17 (May 6, 1988): 261–69.

31. Tatonetti, *Written by the Body*, 142–43.

32. Estrada, "Ojibwe Lesbian Visual AIDS."

33. Tatonetti, *Written by the Body*.

34. Sharon Day, interview by the Tretter Oral History Project, University of Minnesota, 2014.

35. Estrada, "Ojibwe Lesbian Visual AIDS."

36. Chauncey, *Why Marriage?*

37. Katie Batza, Trinity Episcopal Church National Register of Historic Places Registration, 2018, accessed October 7, 2023, https://mostateparks.com/sites/mostateparks/files/TrinityEpiscopalChurch.pdf.

38. Another important development of this phenomenon is homonationalism, which went even further to embrace nationalism as part of LGBTQ identity. It is brought to light in interesting ways in, Ramos and Burnett, "One Out Gay Cop."

39. "The Queer Nation Manifesto," 1990, www.historyisaweapon.com/defcon1/queernation.html.

40. Chris Johnson, "10 Years Later, Firestorm over Gay-Only ENDA Vote Still Informs Movement," *Washington Blade*, November 6, 2017, www.washingtonblade.com/2017/11/06/10-years-later-firestorm-over-gay-only-enda-vote-still-remembered/. Trans people were excluded from the final bill, leaving them open to workplace discrimination with no legal recourse. Instead, battles for trans rights have been waged in courtrooms in a wide array of jurisdictions, creating a patchwork of rights that existed until the Supreme Court decision in June 2020 that transgender workers were protected by a long-standing civil rights law. Adam Liptak, "Civil Rights Law Protects Gay and Transgender Workers, Supreme Court Rules," *New York Times*, June 15, 2020, www.nytimes.com/2020/06/15/us/gay-transgender-workers-supreme-court.html.

41. I want to be careful to point out that many groups, particularly people of color, differently abled people, genderqueer people, and lower-income LGBTQ individuals have had a historically contested relationship with the white, wealthier, and cis LGBTQ movement, and the push for marriage equality simply highlighted and deepened old fissures and cracks.

Conclusion

1. "Missouri Rep. Ian Mackey Confronts Rep. Chuck Basye on Bill That Could Allow Transgender Athletic Bans," KY 3, April 16, 2022, https://www.ky3.com/2022/04/16/missouri-rep-ian-mackey-confronts-rep-chuck-basye-bill-that-could-allow-transgender-athletic-bans/.

2. The geography of these 515 different bills spares no region of the country, and their scope is vast, addressing curriculum changes, access to healthcare, redefinitions of sex, public bathrooms, forced outing in school, barriers to accurate identification, and many more issues. "Mapping Attacks on LGBTQ Rights in U.S. State Legislatures

in 2024," American Civil Liberties Union, www.aclu.org/legislative-attacks-on-lgbtq-rights-2024.

3. "Missouri Rep. Ian Mackey."

4. Natalie Allison, "Guilty Verdict Fuels Trump's Campaign: 'Our Whole Country Is Being Rigged,'" *Politico*, May 30, 2024, https://www.politico.com/news/2024/05/30/trump-campaign-guilty-verdict-trial-00160832.

5. DeSantis, *Courage to Be Free*.

6. Manuel Roig-Franzia, "Ron DeSantis's Scorn-Filled Book Sets the Tone for a Potential Campaign," review of *The Courage to Be Free*, by Ron DeSantis, *Washington Post*, March 2, 2023, https://www.washingtonpost.com/books/2023/02/27/ron-desantis-courage-be-free/.

7. Of course, President George W. Bush initiated the bailout in the days following the 2008 election, leaving the Obama administration with the task of its implementation in the first days of the new administration. Obama's handling of the bailout became an early hallmark of his presidency. David Herszenhorn and David Sanger, "Bush Approves $17.4 Billion Auto Bailout," *New York Times*, December 19, 2008.

8. Joe Biden, "Remarks by President Biden on the Continued Battle for the Soul of the Nation," September 1, 2022, https://www.whitehouse.gov/briefing-room/speeches-remarks/2022/09/01/remarks-by-president-bidenon-the-continued-battle-for-the-soul-of-the-nation/.

9. The White House, "President Biden Announces American Rescue Plan," January 20, 2021, https://www.whitehouse.gov/briefing-room/legislation/2021/01/20/president-biden-announces-american-rescue-plan/.

10. Barbara Sprunt, "Here's What's in the American Rescue Plan," National Public Radio, March 11, 2021, https://www.npr.org/sections/coronavirus-live-updates/2021/03/09/974841565/heres-whats-in-the-american-rescue-plan-as-it-heads-toward-final-passage.

11. "Missouri Rep. Ian Mackey."

12. Moraga and Anzaldua, *This Bridge Called My Back*; Halberstam, *In a Queer Time*; Hill Collins, *Black Feminist Thought*; Bey, *Them Goon Rules*; Morrison, "Home"; Lorde, *Burst of Light*; hooks, *Feminist Theory*.

13. Samuel Bestvater et al., "1. Ten Years of #BlackLivesMatter on Twitter," Pew Research Center, June 29, 2023, https://www.pewresearch.org/internet/2023/06/29/ten-years-of-blacklivesmatter-on-twitter/.

14. "Herstory," Black Lives Matter, accessed June 6, 2024, https://blacklivesmatter.com/about/#our-history.

15. "Timeline of Events in Shooting of Michael Brown in Ferguson," AP News, August 8, 2019, https://apnews.com/article/shootings-police-us-news-st-louis-michael-brown-9aa32033692547699a3b61da8fd1fc62.

16. "About," Black Lives Matter, accessed June 6, 2024, https://blacklivesmatter.com/about/.

17. Evan Hill et al., "How George Floyd Was Killed in Police Custody," New York Times, May 31, 2020, https://www.nytimes.com/2020/05/31/us/george-floyd-investigation.html.

18. Several other murders of Black people occurred at the hands of police or vigilantes during the years since BLM's founding including the more publicized cases of Tamir Rice, Eric Garner, Tanisha Anderson, Mya Hall, Walter Scott, Sandra Bland, and Breonna Taylor.

19. Alim Kheraj, "How Drag Queens Are Going Digital in the Wake of the Coronavirus," *GQ*, March 23, 2020, https://www.gq.com/story/how-drag-queens-are-going-digital-in-the-wake-of-coronavirus; Brittany Spanos, "As Gay Bars Close, Drag Shows Go Online," *Rolling Stone*, March 24, 2020, https://www.rollingstone.com/culture/culture-features/virtual-drag-shows-coronavirus-pandemic-970347/.

20. Sharon Cohen, "Millions of Hungry Americans Turn to Food Banks for 1st Time," AP News, December 7, 2020, https://apnews.com/article/race-and-ethnicity-hunger-coronavirus-pandemic-4c7f1705c6d8ef5bac241e6cc8e331bb; "Thousands of Cars Form Lines to Collect Food in Covid-Hit Texas," *CNN*, November 15, 2020, https://www.cnn.com/2020/11/15/us/dallas-texas-food-bank-coronavirus/index.html.

21. Gobby and Everett, "Policing Indigenous Land Defense"; Gobby and Gareau, "Understanding the Crises."

22. Yessenia Funes, "Fighting Line 3 From a Queer, Indigenous Perspective," Atmos, June 14, 2021, https://atmos.earth/line-3-protests-indigenous-queer-lgbtq/.

23. Zaria Howell, "Indigenous Women and LGBTQ+ People Led Dakota Access Pipeline Protests. Five Years Later, They Reflect on Standing Rock," The 19th, May 20, 2021, https://19thnews.org/2021/05/indigenous-women-and-lgbtq-people-led-dakota-access-pipeline-protests-five-years-later-they-reflect-on-standing-rock/.

Bibliography

Primary Sources

Oral Interviews by the Author

Jim Andris, August 21, 2018.
Brenda Armour, December 11, 2018.
Evelyn Cohen, November 1, 2018.
Philip Deitch, September 12, 2018.
Daniel Flier, January 10, 2019.
Chuck Gulas, December 14, 2018.
Tom Harper, October 2, 2018.
Gary Hirshberg, September 26, 2018.
Cathy Johnson, July 9, 2018.
Jay Johnson, May 9, 2017.
Opal Jones, November 30, 2018.
Sheryl Kelly, March 7, 2019.
Bill LaRock, June 10, 2018.
Mayer and Pat Levy, December 4, 2018.
Keith Price, October 29, 2018.
Michael Slawin, June 12, 2018.
Sister Joann Stuever, February 6, 2019.
Donna Sweet, February 5, 2019.
Jim Thomas, August 27, 2018.
Jim Timmerberg, December 6, 2018.
Erise Williams, May 31, 2018.
Rodney Wilson, July 17, 2018.

Archives

Iowa City, Iowa
   University of Iowa Special Collections
      Barbara Fassbinder Papers
      Emma Goldman Clinic Papers
      Gay, Lesbian, Bisexual, Transgender and Allies Union Records
      Joyce Nielson Papers
      Kathleen Wood Laurila Papers
      Linda Yanney Papers
      Patricia Herring Papers
      University of Iowa News Service Papers

Kansas City, Missouri
   GLAMA Archives, University of Missouri
      AIDS Service Foundation Papers
      Barry Porter Collection
      Bill Todd and Art Bratt Collection
      Larry Sullivan Collection
      Lesbian and Gay Community Center of Kansas City
      Miriam Hennosy Collection
      PFLAG Collection
      Scoop Phillips Collection
      Spirit of Hope MCC Scrapbooks
      Steven R. Pierce Collection
   State Historical Society of Missouri
      Estevez Collection
      Lesbian, Gay, Bisexual, Transgender History Project Papers
      Mayor Vincent Schoemehl Papers
      MCC of Greater St. Louis
      Personal Rights of Missourians (PROMO) Papers
      Privacy Rights Education Project Papers
      St. Louis Lesbian and Gay Archives
Lawrence, Kansas
   University of Kansas Spencer Research Library
      Bruce McKinney Collection
      Dennis Dailey Collection
      Jesse Milan Papers
      Kristi Parker Collection
      Rich Crank Collection
Los Angeles, California
   ONE National Gay and Lesbian Archives
      Laud Humphreys Papers
St. Louis, Missouri
   Missouri History Museum Archives
      AIDS Foundation of St. Louis Records
      Michael Slawin Papers
      Pat and Mayer Levy
      Richard A. Gephardt Campaign Papers
      Richard A. Gephardt Congressional Papers
      St. Louis Effort for AIDS Papers
      St. Louis Gay and Lesbian Community Collection
      Timothy Cusick
   Rodney Wilson, personal archives
   St. Louis Archdiocese Archives
      Administrative Records
      Executive Records
      Historical Records

Washington University Bernard Beck Medical Library Archives
    AIDS Center, WUSM (AIDS Clinical Study Group)
    AIDS Clinic Trials Unit, WUSM
    John William Campbell Collection
    Psychiatry Department Records
    Robert C. Kolodny Collection
    St. Louis Effort for AIDS
    Washington University School of Medicine Papers, 1990–1999
Wichita, Kansas
    Joann Stuever, personal archives

Periodicals

Chicago Tribune
Des Moines Register
Gay News Telegraph
Gazette (Cedar Rapids, IA)
GQ
HIV+ Magazine
Los Angeles Times
Missouri Independent (Jefferson City, MO)
Morbidity and Mortality Weekly Report
New York Native
New York Times
Now
Nursing
Oklahoman (Oklahoma City, OK)
Politico
POZ
Public Health Reports
Rolling Stone
Variety
Washington Blade
Washington Post
Waterloo Courier (Waterloo, IA)
Windy City Times
Wichita Eagle

Secondary Sources

Books

Ahmed, Sara. *Strange Encounters: Embodied Others in Post-Coloniality*. Transformations. New York: Routledge, 2000.

Anderson, Benedict R. *Imagined Communities: Reflections on the Origin and Spread of Nationalism*. Rev. ed. New York: Verso, 2006.

Anzaldúa, Gloria, and AnaLouise Keating, eds. *This Bridge We Call Home: Radical Visions for Transformation*. Edited by Gloria Anzaldúa. New York: Routledge, 2002.

Bailey, Beth L. *Sex in the Heartland*. Cambridge, MA: Harvard University Press, 1999.

Baker, Martha K., and Etta Taylor. *A History of Trinity Church, St. Louis, 1975–2005*. St. Louis, MO: 2005.

Barrett-Fox, Rebecca. *God Hates: Westboro Baptist Church, American Nationalism, and the Religious Right*. Lawrence: University Press of Kansas, 2016.

Baum, L. Frank. *Them Goon Rules: Fugitive Essays on Radical Black Feminism*. Feminist Wire. Tucson: University of Arizona Press, 2019.

———. *The Wizard of Oz*. New York: North-South Books, 1996.Bey, Marquis. *Cistem Failure: Essays on Blackness and Cisgender*. Asterisk. Durham, NC: Duke University Press, 2022. www.jstor.org/stable/10.2307/j.ctv2rr3g52.

Bost, Darius. *Evidence of Being: The Black Gay Cultural Renaissance and the Politics of Violence*. Chicago: University of Chicago Press, 2018.
Branham, Richard L., George F. McCleary, and Lawrence Convention & Visitors Bureau. *Quantrill's Raid: The Lawrence Massacre*. Lawrence, KS: Lawrence Convention and Visitors Bureau, 1997.
Brier, Jennifer. *Infectious Ideas: U.S. Political Responses to the AIDS Crisis*. Chapel Hill: University of North Carolina Press, 2009.
Butler, Judith. *Precarious Life: The Powers of Mourning and Violence*. New York: Verso, 2004.
———. *Undoing Gender*. New York: Routledge, 2004.
Carroll, Tamar W. *Mobilizing New York: AIDS, Antipoverty, and Feminist Activism*. Gender and American Culture. Chapel Hill: University of North Carolina Press, 2015.
Cartwright, Ryan Lee. *Peculiar Places: A Queer Crip History of White Rural Nonconformity*. Chicago: University of Chicago Press, 2021.
Chauncey, George. *Why Marriage? The History Shaping Today's Debate over Gay Equality*. New York: Basic Books, 2004.
Cohen, Cathy J. *The Boundaries of Blackness: AIDS and the Breakdown of Black Politics*. Chicago: University of Chicago Press, 1999.
Connelley, William Elsey. *Quantrill and the Border Wars*. New York: Pageant, 1956.
Crimp, Douglas. *Melancholia and Moralism: Essays on AIDS and Queer Politics*. Cambridge, MA: MIT Press, 2002.
Crimp, Douglas, and Leo Bersani. *AIDS: Cultural Analysis, Cultural Activism*. Cambridge, MA: MIT Press, 1988.
Curtis, Edward. *Muslims of the Heartland: How Syrian Immigrants Made a Home in the American Midwest*. New York: New York University Press, 2022.
Darman, Jonathan. *Landslide: LBJ and Ronald Reagan at the Dawn of a New America*. New York: Random House, 2014.
Deer, Sarah. *The Beginning and End of Rape: Confronting Sexual Violence in Native America*. Minneapolis: University of Minnesota Press, 2015.
D'Emilio, John. *Sexual Politics, Sexual Communities: The Making of a Homosexual Minority in the United States, 1940–1970*. Chicago: University of Chicago Press, 1983.
DeSantis, Ron. *The Courage to Be Free: Florida's Blueprint for America's Revival*. Northampton, MA: Broadside Books, 2023.
Ehrman, John. *The Eighties: America in the Age of Reagan*. New Haven, CT: Yale University Press, 2005.
Fink, Deborah. *Cutting into the Meatpacking Line: Workers and Change in the Rural Midwest*. Studies in Rural Culture. Chapel Hill: University of North Carolina Press, 1998.
Forstie, Clare. *Queering the Midwest: Forging LGBTQ Community*. New York: New York University Press, 2022.
Foucault, Michel. *The Birth of the Clinic: An Archaeology of Medical Perception*. New York: Pantheon, 1973.

———. *Discipline and Punish: The Birth of the Prison*. New York: Pantheon, 1977.
———. *The History of Sexuality*. New York: Vintage Books, 1988.
Frank, Thomas. *What's the Matter with Kansas? How Conservatives Won the Heart of America*. New York: Metropolitan Books, 2004.
Gilmore, Ruth Wilson. *Abolition Geography: Essays Towards Liberation*. Brooklyn, NY: Verso Press, 2022.
———. *Golden Gulag: Prisons, Surplus, Crisis, and Opposition in Globalizing California*. Oakland: University of California Press, 2007.
Griffith, Jane. *Words Have a Past: The English Language, Colonialism, and the Newspapers of Indian Boarding Schools*. Toronto: University of Toronto Press, 2019.
Halberstam, Jack. *In a Queer Time and Place: Transgender Bodies, Subcultural Lives*. New York: New York University Press, 2005.
———. *The Queer Art of Failure*. Durham, NC: Duke University Press, 2011.
———. *Trans: A Quick and Quirky Account of Gender Variability*. Oakland: University of California Press, 2018.
Hall, Stuart. *Essential Essays*. Vol. 1, *Foundations of Cultural Studies*. Durham, NC: Duke University Press, 2019.
Halvorson, Britt E., and Joshua O. Reno. *Imagining the Heartland: White Supremacy and the American Midwest*. Oakland: University of California Press, 2022.
Hamer. Jennifer. *Abandoned in the Heartland: Work, Family, and Living in East St. Louis*. Oakland: University of California Press, 2011.
Hanhardt, Christina B. *Safe Space: Gay Neighborhood History and the Politics of Violence*. Perverse Modernities. Durham, NC: Duke University Press, 2013.
Hayward, Steven F. *The Age of Reagan: The Fall of the Old Liberal Order, 1964–1980*. Roseville, CA: Forum, 2001.
Herring, Scott. *Another Country: Queer Anti-Urbanism*. Sexual Cultures. New York: New York University Press, 2010.
Hill Collins, Patricia. *Black Feminist Thought: Knowledge, Consciousness, and the Politics of Empowerment*. 2nd ed. New York: Routledge, 2009.
Hoganson, Kristin L. *The Heartland: An American History*. New York: Penguin, 2019.
hooks, bell. *Feminist Theory: From Margin to Center*. New York: Routledge, 2015.
Humphreys, Laud. *Out of the Closets: The Sociology of Homosexual Liberation*. Englewood Cliffs, NJ: Prentice-Hall, 1972.
Janovy, C. J. *No Place like Home: Lessons in Activism from LGBT Kansas*. Lawrence: University Press of Kansas, 2018.
Johnson, Haynes. *Sleepwalking through History: America in the Reagan Years*. New York: W. W. Norton, 2003.
Johnson, Victoria E. *Heartland TV: Prime Time Television and the Struggle for U.S. Identity*. New York: New York University Press, 2008.
Jones, Cleve. *When We Rise: My Life in the Movement*. New York: Hachette Books, 2016.
Kowalewski, Mark R. *All Things to All People: The Catholic Church Confronts the AIDS Crisis*. Albany: State University of New York Press, 1994.

Krehbiel, Randy. *Tulsa, 1921: Reporting a Massacre*. Norman: University of Oklahoma Press, 2019.

Krupat, Arnold. *Changed Forever: American Indian Boarding-School Literature*. Native Traces. Albany: State University of New York Press, 2018.

Levenson, Jacob. *The Secret Epidemic: The Story of AIDS in Black America*. Palatine, IL: Anchor, 2005.

Lorde, Audre. *A Burst of Light*. Toronto: Women's Press, 1988.

Lugones, María. *Pilgrimages/Peregrinajes: Theorizing Coalition against Multiple Oppressions*. Lanham, MD: Rowman & Littlefield, 2003.

McKay, Richard A. *Patient Zero and the Making of the AIDS Epidemic*. Chicago: University of Chicago Press, 2017.

Moraga, Cherrie, and Gloria Anzaldúa, eds. *This Bridge Called My Back: Writings by Radical Women of Color*. New York: Kitchen Table, Women of Color Press, 1984.

Moreton, Bethany. *To Serve God and Wal-Mart: The Making of Christian Free Enterprise*. Cambridge, MA: Harvard University Press, 2009.

Morley, David. *Home Territories: Media, Mobility, and Identity*. New York: Routledge, 2000.

Mumford, Kevin. *Not Straight, Not White: Black Gay Men from the March on Washington to the AIDS Crisis*. Illustrated ed. Chapel Hill: University of North Carolina Press, 2016.

Murray, Heather. *Not in This Family: Gays and the Meaning of Kinship in Postwar North America*. Philadelphia: University of Pennsylvania Press, 2010.

Nabhan-Warren, Kristy. *Meatpacking America: How Migration, Work, and Faith Unite and Divide the Heartland*. Chapel Hill: University of North Carolina Press, 2021.

O'Loughlin, Michael J. *Hidden Mercy: AIDS, Catholics, and the Untold Stories of Compassion in the Face of Fear*. Minneapolis, MN: Broadleaf Books, 2021.

Pépin, Jacques. *The Origins of AIDS*. 2nd ed. Cambridge: Cambridge University Press, 2021.

Perlstein, Rick. *Reaganland: America's Right Turn, 1976–1980*. New York: Simon & Schuster, 2020.

Petro, Anthony M. *After the Wrath of God: AIDS, Sexuality, & American Religion*. Illustrated ed. Oxford: Oxford University Press, 2015.

Puar, Jasbir K. *Queer Tourism: Geographies of Globalization*. Durham, NC: Duke University Press, 2001.

———. *Terrorist Assemblages: Homonationalism in Queer Times*. Next Wave. Durham, NC: Duke University Press, 2007.

Renfro, Paul. *The Life and Death of Ryan White: AIDS and Inequality in America*. Chapel Hill: University of North Carolina Press, 2024.

Royles, Dan. *To Make the Wounded Whole: The African American Struggle against HIV/AIDS*. Illustrated ed. Chapel Hill: University of North Carolina Press, 2020.

Schulman, Bruce. *The Seventies: The Great Shift in American Culture, Society, and Politics*. Cambridge, MA: Da Capo Press, 2002.

Schulman, Sarah. *Let the Record Show: A Political History of ACT UP New York, 1987–1993*. New York: Farrar, Straus and Giroux, 2021.

Shilts, Randy. *And the Band Played On: Politics, People, and the AIDS Epidemic.* New York: Penguin, 1988.
Spade, Dean. *Mutual Aid: Building Solidarity during This Crisis.* New York: Verso, 2020.
Stewart-Winter, Timothy. *Queer Clout: Chicago and the Rise of Gay Politics.* Philadelphia: University of Pennsylvania Press, 2015.
Sturken, Marita. *Tangled Memories: The Vietnam War, the AIDS Epidemic, and the Politics of Remembering.* Berkeley: University of California Press, 1997.
Tatonetti, Lisa. *Written by the Body: Gender Expansiveness and Indigenous Non-Cis Masculinities.* Minneapolis: University of Minnesota Press, 2021.
Thrasher, Steven W. *The Viral Underclass: The Human Toll When Inequality and Disease Collide.* New York: Celadon Books, 2022.
Vernon, Irene S. *Killing Us Quietly: Native Americans and HIV/AIDS.* Lincoln: University of Nebraska Press, 2001.
Vider, Stephen. *The Queerness of Home: Gender, Sexuality, and the Politics of Domesticity after World War II.* Chicago: University of Chicago Press, 2021.
Warren, Wilson J. *Tied to the Great Packing Machine: The Midwest and Meatpacking.* Iowa City: University of Iowa Press, 2007.
White, Heather R. *Reforming Sodom: Protestants and the Rise of Gay Rights.* Chapel Hill: University of North Carolina Press, 2015.Wuthnow, Robert. *Red State Religion: Faith and Politics in America's Heartland.* Princeton, NJ: Princeton University Press, 2011.

Journal Articles and Book Chapters

Ayala, George, and Andrew Spieldenner. "HIV Is a Story First Written on the Bodies of Gay and Bisexual Men." *American Journal of Public Health* 111, no. 7 (2021): 1240–42.
Batza, Katie. "Opening DOORWAYS and Closing Others: Tactical Deployments of Respectability, Religion, and Race in St. Louis." In *Resist, Organize, Build: Feminist and Queer Activism in Britain and the United States during the Long 1980s,* edited by Sarah Crook and Charlie Jeffries. Albany: State University of New York Press, 2022.
Bell, Jonathan. "Between Private and Public: AIDS, Health Care Capitalism, and the Politics of Respectability in 1980s America." *Journal of American Studies* (2018): 1–25.
Bell, Jonathan, Darius Bost, Jennifer Brier, Julio Capó Jr., Jih-Fei Cheng, Daniel M. Fox, Christina Hanhardt, Emily K. Hobson, and Dan Royles, "Interchange: HIV/AIDS and U.S. History." *Journal of American History* 104, no. 2 (September 2017): 431–60.
Bhaman, Salonee. "'For a Few Months of Peace': Housing and Care in the Early AIDS Crisis." *Radical History Review* 140 (May 2021): 78–106.
Bost, Darius. "At the Club: Locating early Black gay AIDS Activism in Washington D.C." *Occasion* 8 (2015): 1.
Brier, Jennifer. "Locating Lesbian and Feminist Responses to AIDS, 1982–1984." *Women's Studies Quarterly* 35, no. 1/2 (April 1, 2007): 234–48.

Capozzola, Christopher. "A Very American Epidemic: Memory Politics and Identity Politics in the AIDS Memorial Quilt, 1985–1993." *Radical History Review* 82 (January 2002): 91–109.

Davenport, Doris. "All This, and Honeysuckles Too." In *Bloodroot: Reflections on Place by Appalachian Women Writers*, edited by Joyce Dyer. Louisville: University Press of Kentucky, 1998.

Davis, D. "'Understanding AIDS'—the National AIDS Mailer." *Public Health Reports* 106, no. 6 (1991): 656–62.

D'Emilio, John. "Capitalism and Gay Identity," In *Culture, Society, and Sexuality*, edited by Richard Parker and Peter Aggleto. New York: Routledge, 2007.

Esparza, René. "Black Bodies on Lockdown: AIDS Moral Panic and the Criminalization of HIV in Times of White Injury." *Journal of African American History* 104, no. 2 (March 2019): 250–80.

———. "Great Gay Return: AIDS 'Homecoming' Narratives and Middle America's Fantasies of Racial Reconciliation." Queer History Conference, San Francisco, California, June 2022.

———. "Queering the Homeland: Chicanidad, Racialized Homophobia, and the Political Economy of Homopatriarchy." *Feminist Formations* 29, no. 2 (2017): 147–76.

Estrada, Gabriel. "Ojibwe Lesbian Visual AIDS: On the Red Road with Carole laFavor, *Her Giveaway* (1988), and Native LGBTQ2 Film History." *Journal of Lesbian Studies* 20 (July 1, 2016): 388–407.

Fassbinder, B. "It's Time to Face the Enemy—Together." *Critical Care Nurse* 12, no. 7 (October 1, 1992): 112.

Gobby, Jen, and Lucy Everett. "Policing Indigenous Land Defense and Climate Activism: Learnings from the Frontlines of Pipeline Resistance in Canada." In *Enforcing Ecocide: Power, Policing & Planetary Militarization*, edited by Alexander Dunlap and Andrea Brock. Cham, Switzerland: Springer International, 2022.

Gobby, Jen, and Kristian Gareau. "Understanding the Crises, Uncovering Root Causes, and Envisioning the World(s) We Want: Conversations with the Anti-Pipeline Movements in Canada." In *Routledge Handbook of Climate Justice*, edited by Tahseen Jafry. New York: Routledge, 2018.

Hammonds, Evelynn. "Missing Persons: African American Women, AIDS, and the History of Disease." In *Words of Fire: An Anthology of African American Feminist Thought*, edited by Beverly Guy-Sheftal. New York: New Press, 1995.

Herring, John. "Tribute to Barbara Fassbinder, RN." *Nursing* 25, no. 12 (December 1995): 56.

Herring, Scott. "'Hixploitation' Cinema, Regional Drive-Ins, and the Cultural Emergence of a Queer New Right." *GLQ: A Journal of Lesbian and Gay Studies* 20, no. 1–2 (April 1, 2014): 95–113.

Higby, Toby. "Heartland: The Politics of Regional Signifier." *Middle West Review* 1, no. 1 (Fall 2014): 81–90.

Hobson, Emily K. "The AIDS Quilt in Prison." *Radical History Review* 148 (January 2024): 9–29.

Manalansan, M. F., C. Nadeau, R. T. Rodríguez, and S. B. Somerville. "Queering the Middle." *GLQ: A Journal of Gay and Lesbian Studies* 20, no. 1–2 (2014).

Miller, Joshua H. "Coalitional Fronting and Shared *Ethos* Cultivation in the Case of the Council on Religion and the Homosexual." *Women's Studies in Communication* 44, no. 4 (2021): 542–62.

Montgomery, S. B., J. G. Joseph, M. H. Becker, D. G. Ostrow, R. C. Kessler, and J. P. Kirscht. "The Health Belief Model in Understanding Compliance with Preventive Recommendations for AIDS: How Useful?" *AIDS Education and Prevention: Official Publication of the International Society for AIDS Education* 1, no. 4 (Winter 1989): 303–23.

Morrison, Toni. "Home." In *The House That Race Built: Original Essays by Toni Morrison, Angela Y. Davis, Cornel West, and Others on Black Americans and Politics in America Today*, edited by Wahneema Lubiano. New York: Vintage Books, 1997.

Ramos, Nic John. "Poor Influences and Criminal Locations: Los Angeles's Skid Row, Multicultural Identities, and Normal Homosexuality." *American Quarterly* 71, no. 2 (2019): 541–67.

Ramos, Nic John, and Alex Burnett. "One Out Gay Cop: Gay Moderates, Proposition 64, and Policing in Early AIDS-Crisis Los Angeles, 1969–1992." *Journal of the History of Sexuality* 31, no. 3 (September 2022): 361–93.

Royles, Dan. "'Don't We Die Too?': The Politics of AIDS and Race in Philadelphia." In *Beyond the Politics of the Closet: Gay Rights and the American State since the 1970s*, edited by Jonathan Bell. Philadelphia: University of Pennsylvania Press, 2020.

Rzeznik, Thomas. "The Church and the AIDS Crisis in New York City." *U.S. Catholic Historian* 34, no. 1 (Winter 2016): 143–65.

Testa, Nino. "'If You Are Reading It, I Am Dead': Activism, Local History, and the AIDS Quilt." *Public Historian* 44, no. 3 (August 2022): 24–57.

Wilson, Rodney C. "'The Seed Time of Gay Rights': Rev. Carol Cureton, the Metropolitan Community Church, and Gay St. Louis, 1969–1980." *Gateway Heritage* (Fall 1994): 36.

Index

Italic page numbers refer to illustrations.

activism: AIDS, 46, 50, 115, 117–21; anti-abortion, 42, 112; die-ins, 52, 66; Indigenous AIDS, 115; Indigenous anti-pipeline, 131–32; protests in Midwestern cities, 48; radical approaches to, 48–49, 102. *See also* ACT UP (AIDS Coalition to Unleash Power); political frameworks
ACT UP (AIDS Coalition to Unleash Power), 24, 109, 117; and AIDS Memorial Quilt, 30; Change the Definition campaign, 48; in New York, 66; Omaha chapter, 49; smaller local chapters, 49, 147n10; in St. Louis, 47–51, 63; Stop the Church campaign, 52
Adorers of the Blood of Christ, 96–97
Affordable Care Act (Obamacare), 125
African American communities. *See* Black communities
agriculture: corporate farming and migrant work, 19; family farms, 18; migrant farm labor, 27
Ahalya Project (Tulsa, OK), 41
Ahmed, Sara, 12
AIDS. *See* HIV/AIDS epidemic
AIDS activism: and burnout, 46; heartland ideals used in, 117–21; Indigenous, 115; and Midwestern values, 50
"AIDS Comes to a Small Town" (*Oprah* episode), 22
AIDS House (Wichita, KS), 96–99
AIDS phobia, 35, 43–44
AIDS prevention and educational efforts, 86–87, 90
AIDS Quilt, 29–30, 37, 47, 49–50; criticism of, 30

Allen, John, 62
Allen, Michael, 63–64, 67
American Academy of HIV Medicine Specialists, 80, 82
American Civil Liberties Union (ACLU), 60
And the Band Played On (Shilts), 22–23
anti-abortion activism, 42, 112
Anzaldúa, Gloria, 33–34
ARC (AIDS-related complex), 34
Ashcroft, John, 106
assimilationism, 102, 118, 121
Atchison, KS, 83
AZT (drug treatment), 24, 38, 108

Bacon, Kevin, 14, 14–15
Bailey, Beth, 3
ballroom culture, 146n26
Basye, Stephen, 122–23
Baum, L. Frank, 12
B-Boy Blues (Hardy), 89
B-Boy Festival, 89–90
Bell, Jonathan, 23
belonging, sense of, 29, 33, 35, 36–37, 44, 46, 55, 88–90, 91
A Better Family Life, 88
Bewick, Charles, 63
Bey, Marquis, 12
Bhaman, Salonee, 23
Big Wind (Standing Rock organizer), 131
binary frameworks, 12
Black communities: Black churches, 69; Black joy, 128; free Black settlement in Reconstruction era, 20; responses to HIV/AIDS in, 85–93; women with HIV/AIDS in, 32
Black feminist theory, 127

Black Lives Matter (BLM) movement, 128–30, 132
Black Pride Festival, 90
Blacks Assisting Blacks against AIDS (BABAA), 86–93, 107, 117
Blake, Sir Bobby, 92
blood transfusions, 111. *See also* White, Ryan
Bost, Darius, 23, 69, 88
Bowers v. Hardwick, 63, 105
Boys Don't Cry (film), 21
bridging, 34, 65
Brier, Jennifer, 23
Brown, Michael, 128
buddy programs, 107
Bureau of Indian Affairs, 40
Bush, George W., 91, 106
Byrd, James, Jr., 21

"Called to Compassion and Responsibility" (pastoral statement), 66–67
capitalism, 17, 125. *See also* neoliberalism
caregiving and mutual aid, 44, 129–30
Carrol, Tamar, 23
Cartwright, Ryan, 12
Castile, Philando, 128
Catholic Church: and AIDS activists, 65; anti-condom stance of, 99; "Called to Compassion and Responsibility" (pastoral statement), 66–76; Catholic-affiliated hospitals, 93, 96; *Many Faces of AIDS, The* (pastoral statement), 65–66; nuns' role in AIDS response, 96–99; response of to AIDS, 52; in St. Louis, 56–57
CDC (Centers for Disease Control), 24, 93; *Morbidity and Mortality Weekly Report (MMWR)*, 25; "Understanding AIDS" mass mailing, 114
Cemetery, February 1991 (Evans), 100
Change the Definition campaign (ACT UP), 48
Chapman, Bill, 61, 63, 123

Chauncey, George, 118
Cherokee Nation, 40. *See also* Native American populations
Chicana feminist theory, 33
Christ Church Cathedral, 67
church youth groups, 55
Civil War, 19
class division, erasure of, 17
Clement, Beth, 12
Clinton, Bill, 105, 114
closeted identities, 71, 95
coastal gay communities: collapse of, 45; focus on, 23–24, 124
Cohen, Cathy, 23, 69, 88
colonialism, 31; erasure of, 15
"coming home syndrome," 26, 30–31, 81–82. *See also* homecomings
condom distribution, 67, 91, 106–7; Catholic anti-condom stance, 99; safe sex education, 99
ConnectCare, 97
conservatism: anti-elitism, 17; New Right, 117; and Religious Right, 54–55
Cooper, Lynn, 68
Costner, Kevin, 14
The Courage to Be Free (DeSantis), 124
COVID-19 pandemic, 126, 129–30
Crimp, Douglas, 32
Cullors, Patrisse, 128
culture wars, 1–2

Dakota Access pipeline, 131–32
Darnell, Ian, 59, 61
Daughters of Bilitis, 50
Davenport, Doris, 12, 33
Day, Sharon, 116
Deep Creek Road, Flint Hills, KS, 1979 (Iversen), 10
Delaware Nation, 40. *See also* Native American populations
Deleuze, Gilles, 9
D'Emilio, John, 45
Derrida, Jacques, 32

DeSantis, Ron, 124
die-ins, 52, 66
Dignity (Catholic LGBTQ group), 65
DOORWAYS (housing organization), 43–44, 56, 64–73, 107–8, 109, 117
Dust Bowl, 20–21

Edland, Michael, 43
education, 110–17; AIDS prevention, 86–87, 90, 111–12; for Native populations, 115; safe-sex, 106–7, 112–13; and Donna Sweet, 111–14
EFA. *See* St. Louis Effort for AIDS (EFA)
Elders, Jocelyn, 105
"elites," 124
Emmanuel Episcopal Church (Webster Groves, MO), 64
Employment Non-Discrimination Act (2007), 120
Empty Train Cars in Wheat Field near Friend, Kansas (Schwarm), 103
Evans, Terry, 10–11, *11*, 12, *13*, 100, 127

Fassbinder, Barbara, 110–11, 113–14, 117
feminist theory, 33
Fent's Prairie, Salina, Kansas (Evans), *13*, 127
Ferguson, MO, 128
fetal HIV, 41
Field of Dreams (film), 14
Finney, Joan, 41
Flier, Daniel, 5, 62, 106–7
"floating signifiers," 32, 34
Florida, 124
Floyd, George, 128
Food and Drug Administration (FDA), 93
Footloose (film), 14, *14–15*
Forstie, Clare, 46, 141n39
4H disease, 34–35
Frank, Thomas, 17

Garden City, KS, 19, 21, 83
Garland, Judy, 29
Garza, Alicia, 128

Gay and Lesbian Students of Kansas (GLSOK), 37
"gay cancer," 34
gay chain migration, 70–71
Gay Liberation Front, 61
Gay Men's Health Crisis, 24, 27, 130
gene editing, 94
Gilmore, Ruth Wilson, 102
Grandberry, Virgil, 86, 88
Grand Island, NE, 19
Graves, Bill, 41–42
Great Migration, 19, 58
GRID (gay-related immune deficiency), 34
Guattari, Félix, 9
Gulas, Chuck, 46

HAART (highly active antiretroviral therapy), 24–25
Halberstam, J., 12
Hall, Stuart, 32
Hammonds, Evelynn, 32
Hanhardt, Christina B., 62
Harambee community center, 90–91
Hardy, James Earl, 89
Harris, Kamala, 125–26
Haskell Indian Nations University, 20, 37–38, 39–40, 41. *See also* Native American populations
hate crimes, 21
"health sovereignty," 116
"heartland": definitions and boundaries of, 9–10, 124; diversity within, 12; erasure of groups ub, 21–23; erasure of HIV/AIDS epidemic in, 22–23, 26; landscapes and topography of, 10, 10–12, *11*; reality of, 18–21; slavery in, 19; as white imaginary, 13–17. *See also* Midwest; white heartland imaginary
Her Giveaway (film), 115
Herring, Scott, 12, 22, 45
Heying, Philip, 79
Hillbilly Elegy (Vance), 126

Index   165

HIV/AIDS epidemic: case numbers in Midwest, 26; CD_4 counts, 48; changes in disease progression, 34; confidentiality rights, 63; criminalization of HIV status, 106; definitions of, 48; dehumanization of victims, 113; emergence of, 1–2; fetal HIV, 41; history of in Midwest, 23–28; HIV testing, 90, 91; and homosexuals, 1; origin stories of, 25–26; pattern of spread in United States, 3; pediatric cases of, 41; response in US Midwest vs. bicoastal response, 3–4; rural landscapes' impact on response, 100–101; vaccine trials, 94–95
hixploitation films, 22
Hobson, Emily, 23
"home": as contested space, 51; creation of, 5; definitions and concepts of, 29, 30–31, 33–37; denial and loss of, 50–51; as domestic space, 35; Earth as, 131–132; homelessness and home recreation, 31–33; imaginary vs. real, 34; material vs. discursive aspects of, 35–36; in Midwest, 31–32; for Native Americans, 40; reimagining, 38, 128–29; and religion's role, 55; renegotiated definitions of by Summer of Mercy, 112–13; safety and lack of safety in, 33–34; and sense of belonging, 36–37; singular vs. systemic levels, 31
"Home" (Morrison), 18
homecoming, 45–46; family reception, 45–46; and funding under Ryan White CARE ACT, 113. See also "coming home syndrome"
homelessness, 41; definitions of, 33; discursive, 42, 139–40n2; nonprofit shelters for unhoused, 43–44; physical vs. emotional, 33
homonationalism, 118, 149n38
homophobia: in Midwest, 35, 98; and religion, 52, 59, 61; and Westboro Baptist Church, 73–76
hospice placements, 38

hospitals: hospital and clinic infrastructures, 93–99; university-affiliated vs. religious group-affiliated, 93–94
House Subcommittee on Health and Environment, 110
housing: discrimination, 106; religious-based coalitions, 67–68
Houska, Angela, 97
Hughes, Langston, 20
Human Rights Campaign (HRC), 109
Humboldt, NE, 21

identity formation: closeted identities, 71, 95; identity-based communities, 50–51; lesbian identities, 114–15; two-spirit people, 115, 131
independence as ideal, 78–79
Indian Health Service, 33, 40; distrust of, 40–41
Indian nations, 39–41. See also Native American populations
Indian reservations, 14
Indigenous AIDS activism, 115
Indigenous people, 14; anti-pipeline activism, 131–32. See also Native American populations
individualism: challenges to, 90; and self-sustainability, 129
innocent vs. guilty binary, 111
intersectionality and Black gay culture, 89–90
Iversen, Earl, 10, 52

John Paul II (pope), 65
Johnson, Cathy, 47–51
Johnson, Colin, 12
Johnson, Jay, 37–42, 76
Jones, Cleve, 50

Kansas: Department of Education, 111, 114; Department of Health, 41; as "free state," 20; Governor's Task Force on AIDS, 111–12; Kansas City ACT UP chapter, 49; medical infrastructure, 27; in white imaginary, 15, 16

Kaposi's sarcoma, 25
Kaya Malaika building, 70
Kelly, Sheryl, 83, 84
Kickapoo Nation, 39. *See also* Native American populations
Kramer, Larry, 23–24

Lacan, Jacques, 32
laFavor, Carole, 114–17, 132
Laramie, WY, 21
LaRock, Bill, 47–51
Latinx feminist theory, 33, 127
Latinx migrants, 19, 83
Lawrence, KS, 3, 4; lynching of Black persons in, 20; Quantrill's Raid, 20
lesbian identities, 114–15
Lévi-Strauss, Claude, 32
LGBTQ equality, 63
LGBTQ History Month, 95
lobbying groups, 105–6
lynching, 20
Lyon, Phyllis, 50

Mackey, Ian, 122–23, 126
MAGA political movement, 124
Mama Nyumba building, 70
Mandrake Society, 60
Manifest Destiny, 15
Many Faces of AIDS, The (pastoral statement), 65–66
marriage: benefits of, 118; equality, 125; same-sex, 118–20, 125, 145n74
Martin, Trayvon, 128
May, John L., 65–67, 108
meatpacking industry, 19, 27
medical care, 78–101; for Black community, 85–93; and discrimination against HIV positive persons, 38; home visits, 84–85; hospital and clinic infrastructures, 93–99; Native American medical traditions, 116; risks and safety for personnel, 110–111; Donna Sweet's work in, 79–86

Midwest: during Civil War, 20; diversity in, 5–6; migration, 19; in popular culture, 14–15; rural landscapes' impact on AIDS response in, 100–101; spread of AIDS in, 3. *See also* "heartland"
migrant farm labor, 27
migration: to coastal communities during pandemic, 46–47; gay chain, 70–71; Great Migration, 19, 58; Latinx migrants, 19; leaving and coming home, 30; regional, 30–31, 45; in Midwest, 20–21
military funerals, protests at, 74–75
militias, white, 21
Miller, J. H., 62
Minnesota American Indian AIDS Task Force, 115
Minority AIDS Initiative, 146n30
Missouri: criminalization of HIV status in, 106; slavery in, 20
Morbidity and Mortality Weekly Report (CDC), 25
Morrison, Toni, 12, 18
mutual aid and caregiving, 44, 129–30, 132

NAMES Project, 47, 49
National Conference of Catholic Bishops, 65, 66–67
National HIV Prevention Conference, 90
National Institutes of Health (NIH), 93
nationalism, 75
National Native American AIDS Prevention Center (NNAPC), 39–41
Native American populations, 114–15; anti-pipeline activism of, 131–32; erasure of, 19–20; forced relocation of, 18; Haskell Indian Nations University, 20, 37–38, 39–40, 41; health sovereignty of, 116; HIV/AIDS, 140n18; Indian Health Service, 33, 40–41; medical traditions of, 116; Native AIDS organizations, 115; Native nations, 14, 39–41; Native sovereignty, 116–17; reservations, 27
Nebraska (Springsteen album), 18

Index 167

neoliberalism, 1–2; and individualism and self-sustainability, 129; and "organized abandonment," 102; and responses to AIDS, 102; and self-sufficiency, 44; and social safety net, 93; in US healthcare system, 115; values of, 31
New Right, 117
New York Native (newspaper), 23–24
Nicodemus, KS, 20
No Place like Home (Janovy), 145n74
nostalgia, 32, 35
nuns, 96–99. *See also* Catholic Church
nursing home placements, 38

Obama administration, 124–25
Obamacare (Affordable Care Act), 125
O'Connor, Cardinal John, 52, 66–67
Ojibwe nation, 114. *See also* Native American populations
Operation Rescue, 74
Operation Rescue National (ORN), 112
opportunistic infections, 24, 48
The Oprah Winfrey Show (television series), 22
oral traditions, 115
OUTsmart (newsletter), 105–6

palliative care, 97–99
Paris Is Burning (film), 146n26
Parker, Charlie, 20
personal protective equipment (PPE), 110
Phelps, Fred, 74–76
Pittsburg, KS, 83
political frameworks, 102–21; and education, 110–17; and heartland ideals, 117–21; and lobbying, 105–6; 2024 presidential campaign, 125–26
populism, 17
Positively Native, 115
poverty: erasure of in heartland imaginary, 17–18; neoliberal values and blame, 2
Praying Hands Monument, Graveyard, Route 54 (Iversen), 53

President's Advisory Council for HIV/AIDS, 114
prevention and education, 86–87, 90, 111–12
privacy: concept of, 103–4; rights, 63, 106, 109
Privacy Rights Education Project (PREP), 63, 105–6; *OUTsmart* (newsletter), 105–6; and privacy rights, 109; white heartland ideals, 109
PROMO (Promoting Missouri), 63, 105
prophylactic use. *See* condom distribution
Protestantism, 54

Quantrill's Raid, 20
Queering the Midwest (Forstie), 141n39
Queer Nation, 120
The Queerness of Home (Vider), 35

racial issues: Blacks Assisting Blacks against AIDS (BABAA), 86–93, 107, 117; erasure of, 18–19; segregation in St. Louis, 87
racism: erasure of in heartland, 17; and HIV/AIDS as tool for blame, 2
Ramos, Nic John, 23
Rayford, Robert, 25, 26
Reagan, Ronald, 18, 24, 54; neoliberal values, 31, 33
Reagan administration, 117
redlining, 20
religion, 52–77; Black churches, 69; "blame and shame," culture of, 71–72; bridge-building, 65; diversity in responses to AIDS, 55–56; and homophobia, 52; interdenominational coalitions, 68–69, 108; and nationalism, 75; Protestantism, 54; role of in Heartland AIDS response, 52–58; sexuality, spiritual explorations of, 61. *See also* Catholic Church
Religious Right, 1, 54–55
Repurposed Billboard West of Salina, Kansas (Heying), 79

respectability: politics, 65, 91; as tool, 61–62, 72–73
rights: privacy, 63, 106, 109; privacy vs. LGBT, 106
Ross, Mary, 70
Royles, Daniel, 23, 69, 88
rurality: and healthcare, 82, 84, 93, 100; hixploitation films, 22; landscape's impact on AIDS response, 11, 100–101; and regional migration, 44–45; role in shaping heartland, 9. *See also* agriculture
Rustin, Bayard, 93
Rustin Center, 93
Ryan White CARE Act (1990), 41, 84, 107, 113

safe-sex education, 106–7, 112–13
safe-sex parties, 91–92
Safe Space (Hanhardt), 62
Salina, KS, 83
same-sex marriage, 118–20, 145n74; Supreme Court decision, 125
San Francisco Council on Religion and the Homosexual (CRH), 62
Schulman, B. J., 13
Schulman, Sarah, 23
Schwarm, Larry, 103
secrecy, 47; closeted identities, 71, 95; and sense of unbelonging, 36–37
sense of belonging, 29, 33, 35, 36–37, 44, 46, 55, 88–90, 91
sex education, 111–12; abstinence-only, 112
Sex in the Heartland (Bailey), 3
sexuality, spiritual exploration of, 61
Shanti Project, 52–53
Shepard, Matthew, 21
signifiers, floating, 32, 34
Sisco, Mike, 22
Sisters of Perpetual Indulgence, 50. *See also* Catholic Church
slaughterhouses, 19
slavery, 19–20
Smith, Mona, 115

social safety nets: erosion of under neoliberalism, 93; replacement of by religion, 54
Social Security Administration disability benefits, 48
sodomy laws, 105. *See also Bowers v. Hardwick*
Somali migrants, 19, 21
Somerville, Siobahn, 12
sovereignty, 116–17
space: creation of "home," 5; "home" as domestic space, 35; "home" as safe space, 33–34; "in-between" spaces, 12. *See also* "home"
Spirits Alive, 115
Springsteen, Bruce, 18
S. P. v. Sullivan, 48
Standing Rock protests (2016), 131–32
Sterling, Alton, 128
St. Louis, MO: ACT UP St. Louis, 47–51; AIDS epidemic response, 62–63; background and overview of, 56–58; Blacks Assisting Blacks against AIDS (BABAA), 86–93; DOORWAYS (housing organization), 43–44, 56, 64–73; racial dividing lines, 43, 59, 87; Trinity Episcopal Church, 56, 58–64
St. Louis Effort for AIDS (EFA), 47, 48, 62–63, 106–9, 117, 130
St. Louis Metropolitan Community Church (MCC), 94–96
St. Louis University, 94, 107; community action board (CAB), 95
Stop the Church campaign (ACT UP), 52
St. Patrick's Cathedral, New York City, 66
Stuever, Sister Joann, 5, 97–99
Sturken, Marika, 49–50
Summer of Mercy (1991), 42, 112
Sweet, Donna, 36, 45, 79–86, 17; and AIDS House hospice facility, 97; educational work of, 111–14

Tatonetti, Lisa, 114
Teena, Brandon, 21

Terraced Plowing with Grass Waterway, April 1991 (Evans), 11
Terry, Randall, 74
This Bridge We Call Home (Anzaldúa), 33–34
A Thousand Plateaus (Deleuze and Guattari), 9
Thrasher, Steven, 17–18
Tiller, George, 148n23
Tometi, Opal, 128
Topeka, KS: ACT UP chapter, 49; Topeka AIDS Project, 37–42, 96; Westboro Baptist Church, 73–76
transgender populations, 120–21, 149n40; violence against, 21; youth athletic bans, 122–23
Trinity Episcopal Church (St. Louis, MO), 56, 58–64, 123; and same-sex marriage, 119–20
Trump, Donald J., 124
Tucker, George, 64
Tulsa Race Massacre, 20
two-spirit identities, 115, 131

"Understanding AIDS" (CDC mass mailing), 114
unhoused persons. *See* homelessness
United Methodist Mexican American Ministries, 83
University of Kansas, 94; Gay and Lesbian Students of Kansas (GLSOK), 37; liberal environment of, 37–38
University of Nebraska, 94

vaccine trials, 94–95
Valentino, Vicky, 89
Vance, J. D., 125–26
Vider, Stephen, 35
violence: hate crimes, 21; racial, erasure of, 18–19
Viral Underclass, The (Thrasher), 17–18
voter intimidation, 20

Walz, Tim, 125–26
Washington University (St. Louis, MO), 94, 107

Westboro Baptist Church, 56, 73–76
Wetta, Teresa, 97
What's the Matter with Kansas? (Frank), 17
White, Ryan, 110, 111
white heartland imaginary, 35; competing versions of, 123–24; and native sovereignty, 116; efforts to subvert, 61–62; erasure of marginalized people in, 87, 115; "home" in, 67–68; ideals, tactical deployment of, 106–7, 117–21; independence as ideal of, 78–79, 79; opposition to, 115–16; political frameworks of, 108–9; political influence of, 117–21; power o, 49; privacy as ideal of, 104; in 2024 presidential campaign, 125–26; Donna Sweet's use of, 85–86; as tool for education, 110–11; use of religiosity, 54–55; work ethic in heartland imaginary, 14, 15. *See also* "heartland"
whiteness: non-Southern, 13–17, 14, 16; white settler colonialism, 31
Wichita, KS, 94; AIDS House hospice facility, 96–99; Women's Health Care Services, 148n23. *See also* Sweet, Donna
Williams, Erise, 4–5, 86–93, 97
Williams and Associates health center, 93, 117
Williamson, WV, 22
Wilson, Rodney, 94–95
Winfrey, Oprah, 22
Wizard of Oz, The (film), 12, 29–30
women: HIV/AIDS definitions, 24; HIV-positive women, 43–44, 69, 114
Women's Health Care Services (Wichita, KS), 148n23
Wonderful Wizard of Oz, The (Baum), 12

youth: sex education for, 111–12; transgender athletic bans, 122–23
Youth of America, 61

Zimmerman, George, 128

www.ingramcontent.com/pod-product-compliance
Lightning Source LLC
Chambersburg PA
CBHW031447160426
43195CB00010BB/887